W9-AUB-979

THE BASIC CAUSES
OF MODERN DISEASES
AND HOW TO REMEDY THEM

BY HANNA KROEGER

Please visit the Hay House Website at: **www.hayhouse.com**

THE BASIC CAUSES
OF MODERN DISEASES
AND HOW TO REMEDY THEM

Hanna Kroeger

Hay House, Inc.
Carlsbad, CA

Copyright © 1984 by Hanna Kroeger
Revised copyright © 1998

Published and distributed in the United States by:
Hay House, Inc., P.O. Box 5100, Carlsbad, CA 92018-5100
(800) 654-5126 • (800) 650-5115 (fax)

Edited by: Gretchen Lalik of Kroeger Herb Products; and Jill Kramer and Christine Watsky of Hay House • *Designed by:* Wendy Lutge

All rights reserved. No part of this book may be reproduced by any mechanical, photographic, or electronic process, or in the form of a phonographic recording; nor may it be stored in a retrieval system, transmitted, or otherwise be copied for public or private use—other than for "fair use" as brief quotations embodied in articles and reviews without prior written permission of the publisher.

The author of this book does not dispense medical advice or prescribe the use of any technique as a form of treatment for physical or medical problems without the advice of a physician, either directly or indirectly. The intent of the author is only to offer information of a general nature to help you in your quest for emotional and spiritual well-being. In the event you use any of the information in this book for yourself, which is your constitutional right, the author and the publisher assume no responsibility for your actions.

Library of Congress Cataloging-in-Publication Data

Kroeger, Hanna.
    [God helps those who help themselves]
    The basic causes of modern diseases—and how to remedy them / Hanna Kroeger.
        p.   cm.   ISBN 1-56170-527-6 (pbk.)
    1. Holistic medicine. 2. Diseases—Causes and theories of causation. I. Title.
    R733.K676   1998
    616—dc21   98-9733
                                                  CIP

First Published in 1984 by Hanna Kroeger Publications, Boulder, Colorado, under the title
God Helps Those Who Help Themselves

ISBN 1-56170-527-6

01 00 99 98   4 3 2 1
First Printing, Revised Edition, November 1998

Printed in the United States of America

I dedicate this book to
the protector of America, St. Michael,
and to his army of Torchbearers.
— Hanna Kroeger

❧ CONTENTS ❧

⚜ INTRODUCTION ⚜

*"The future belongs to those nations who are willing and capable to adopt the
science of nutrition, and take full advantage of its teachings."*
— Dr. G. von Wendt (Sweden)

What Is Holistic Health?

Webster's *Third International Dictionary* defines *holistic* as "emphasizing the organic or functional relation between parts and wholes, rather than an atomistic approach." In relation to health, this means recognizing that all disease processes involve the whole person. Within the physical dimension, disease in one system of the body affects the other systems. Similarly, imbalance in any one dimension of existence—physical, mental, spiritual, or social—affects the other dimensions.

One reason holistic health is hard to pin down is that it represents an attitude toward health and healing, rather than specific treatments, therapies, or things to do. This attitude is one that emphasizes wellness, preventive care, the responsibility of each of us for our own well-being, and the need to recognize that we are not just a collection of mechanical parts, but an integrated system with physical, mental, spiritual, and social aspects that function in a holistic way.

What is holistic health? You hear the term a lot these days, but few people seem to know what it means. As Dr. Norman Shealy, president of the American Holistic Medical Association, says, "Holistic medicine is like God. You can't quite put your finger on it…it's everywhere…and everything."

Fran Atkinson tells us, "This is Wholism: living each moment and experience to the hilt, with full mind awareness, spirit awareness; letting oneself be washed and cleansed by the pure stream of thankfulness and appreciation."

And Jesus said, "I make you whole," which means all facilities of all dimensions together. The physical body is dependent on your emotional faculties, and your mental outlook is the watchtower.

How to Perform Your Own Miracle Healing

Health balances all aspects of your being—physical, mental, and spiritual. You can manage and balance your own household, you do fine in your own business, you manage and balance your environment, you balance your checkbook, but when it comes to balancing your health, you often let someone else do it. Why? Because you shy away from the work it takes to balance your body chemistry. When it comes to your own thinking and emotions, you quit and go to a psychiatrist, a counselor, your minister, your friends, the card reader, the palm reader, the tea-leaf reader, or the crystal-ball gazer, even though you yourself could do a much better job. Of course, you need tools to do so, and this book will give you those tools. The daring is yours, the work is yours, the determination is yours, but God is with those who help themselves, and the Lord is with you.

There are seven fundamental causes of illness in the spiritual and emotional realm and seven causes in the physical realm. Usually they are not clear-cut. They are interwoven, and one has to diligently undo the many knots one by one to bring back balance. *Balance* is the key word in nature, and *balance* is the key word in health.

❧ CHAPTER ONE ❧

Neglect As a Cause of Ill Health

Neglect is one of the seven physical causes of ill health, and we all neglect our bodies' needs. It is our fault that we do not educate ourselves about the "stuff" we are made of. Did we have our daily vitamins today? Did we do deep inhaling and exhaling? Did we sleep enough? All of these things are essential, and we are the ones who decide whether to neglect our bodies and become a burden to our beloved ones or whether to do our part to stay well.

This is what the self-care movement is all about. Seven hundred courses of self-help are being given in at least 40 states. The self-care movement has grown in a period when a skeptical public is challenging all authorities, including physicians. The self-care movement suggests that we learn the risks of our particular ways of living so we can make sensible changes.

The question comes to mind: Does self-help work? Yes, it does. A tooth is extracted, then starts to bleed. A trip to the emergency room costs $75. A tea bag costs only a few cents. Learning how to use the tea bag rather than the trip to the emergency room will save money and time. We also gain a feeling of confidence from knowing how to take responsibility for ourselves. Most busy physicians encourage us to practice self-care. For the body to be healthy, we have to take care of it daily. Since you usually act as your own doctor anyway, why not learn how to do a good job of it? We all understand that there are situations in which we need surgical and medical help. But take responsibility for your wellness—not sickness—by learning all you can about your body and its care.

Minerals

Before there were vitamins, before there was food, before there was life, there were minerals. Minerals are the real stuff we are made of, and they act as building blocks to all cells in our bodies. The following minerals all play an important part in maintaining health.

Calcium: Calcium is a valuable mineral for the growing person and is of great benefit to those recovering from illnesses. The bones of the body are mainly composed of calcium, and this element gives tone to the muscles, while lack of it leads to decay in the bones and teeth. The human body contains more calcium than any other mineral, over 90 percent of which is deposited in bones and teeth to keep them strong and hard. The remainder is essential for healthy blood, a regular heartbeat, and a healthy nervous system. Calcium deficiency is generally characterized by muscle cramps, numbness, and tingling in arms and legs. Extra calcium is a highly regarded treatment for osteoporosis, arthritis, and rheumatism.

Adequate calcium provides the following benefits:

- Strength and energy
- Decision-making skill
- Invention and good thought production

Inadequate calcium can cause the following problems:

- Stuttering
- Stammering
- Prolapses
- Sores
- Inferiority complex
- Soft bones
- Sore tissue

Calcium cannot be absorbed if iodine is missing.

Zinc: Commonly known zinc benefits often overshadow the mineral's other important duties. It is vital in the absorption and action of many vitamins. It is a component of insulin and necessary for proper skin, nail, and hair growth and appearance. Zinc is also crucial for the speedy, healthy healing of cuts and burns.

The following symptoms may indicate zinc deficiency:

- Stretch marks on the skin
- White spots on the fingernails
- Impaired sexual functioning
- Fatigue
- Prolonged healing of wounds

Zinc is needed for hearing and brain functioning, and is essential for diabetics.

Chromium: A trace mineral whose daily requirements have just recently been recognized, chromium has a crucial role to play in human health. Chromium is responsible for the metabolism of glucose into energy and can boost the effectiveness of insulin. A lack of chromium can result in fatigue, energy loss, and blood sugar imbalance; and symptoms of hypoglycemia, hyperglycemia, and diabetes can also appear. Chromium is routinely deficient in modern American diets, and since we absorb less as we grow older, maintaining proper levels becomes very difficult.

Copper: Copper is necessary for proper iron absorption, bone growth and health, and the production of RNA in the body's cells. Deficiencies are rare, but a lack of copper can cause anemia and edema. On the other hand, since copper competes with zinc in the body, too much copper can precipitate a zinc deficiency.

Iodine: Iodine is required for the proper functioning of the thyroid gland. Iodine plays a major role in regulating the production of energy and stimulating the rate of metabolism. Iodine deficiencies may lead to obesity, sluggishness, slowed mental reactions, and hardening of the arteries.

Magnesium: Magnesium is a powerful agent in the elimination of waste matter from the system. Magnesium deficiencies are quite common. The symptoms include nervousness, muscle twitches, confusion, and the formation of calcium deposits. Because of its importance within the central nervous system, magnesium has a reputation as a calming, relaxing substance.

Iron: Iron carries oxygen from the lungs to all parts of the body. It gives strength to the nerves and muscles and makes the blood rich and pure. Deficiencies commonly include such symptoms as chronic fatigue, pale complexion, constipation, hair loss, and anemia.

Sodium: Sodium is a necessary constituent of the gastric juices and is found in all fluids in the body. It is valuable for general elimination of acids from the system. Sodium keeps other minerals soluble in blood, and it is involved in muscle expansion and contraction. Most people get too much sodium, which can cause dizziness, water retention, and the loss of potassium.

Potassium: Potassium generates the electric and magnetic forces in the body necessary for rebuilding tissues, flesh, bones, and muscles. It gives flexibility to the muscles. Potassium promotes normal growth, helps regulate the heartbeat, and encourages the kidneys to flush out body wastes. Symptoms of deficiency include heart problems, poor reflexes, edema, dry skin, and poor muscle tone. Supplemental potassium can balance out excess salt, lower high blood pressure, reduce blood sugar levels, and relieve water retention.

Manganese: As an enzyme activator and catalyst, manganese provides nourishment to the nerves and brain. A deficiency can prevent the removal of excess sugar from the blood, impair muscle coordination, and cause fatigue and female disorders.

Phosphorus: Phosphorus is a stimulant to the nerves and brain. Without this element, the bones deteriorate, and lung tissues fall prey to infections that under healthy conditions are destroyed by phosphoric acid.

Silicon: Silicon absorbs gases in the body, especially in the bowels, and is a substance in the cells of connective tissues. Silicon is needed for vitamin B assimilation.

Selenium: Selenium has been the subject of much recent interest and favorable publicity. It is highly valued for its natural antioxidant powers, and it is known to retard aging and help preserve tissue elasticity by neutralizing harmful oxidative reactions in the cells. Research into selenium's benefits indicates that it can be helpful in inhibiting tumor formation and heart disease. The main deficiency symptom is premature aging, but deficiencies have also been linked to infertility and lowered intelligence. In spite of its importance to health, many American's are selenium deficient.

Two Kinds of Minerals: Organic and Inorganic

The body is composed of both organic and inorganic elements, and the organic predominates. The organic cannot function properly without the inorganic. Dr. William A. Albrecht, Professor Emeritus of Soils, College of Agriculture, University of Missouri, has devoted a lifetime to research on trace minerals in soil and their effects on plants, animals, and people. He indicates that although some minerals are insoluble (inorganic), they become soluble upon coming in contact with the mucous membranes of the body.

Thus, according to Dr. Albrecht, the insoluble can become available through the exchange transformation to water and can then become available as nourishment. He adds that natural plant growth emphasizes the fact that the inorganic (insoluble), as well as the highly organic (soluble), are both biochemically active. Dr. Albrecht also indicates that chelation may explain why nature can transform an insoluble element into a biochemically active one.

Any biochemistry textbook will tell you that both organic and inorganic elements occur in the body, and both are needed to rebuild the constant wear and tear and degeneration of the body. Phosphorus, for instance, is not only present in inorganic combinations (such as bones, teeth, and blood), but in many organic combinations as well. Inorganic and organic elements are in equilibrium with each other and come from the food we eat and the beverages we drink. In addition, many enzymes require small quantities of inorganic elements for their activity.

Inorganic minerals are needed for your electromagnetic body as well as for building and rebuilding bones, tissues, and the entire you.

Only 4 or 5 percent of the body is composed of minerals (the rest is mostly water), but this small percentage is really vital. Minerals make our teeth and bones hard and give shape and function to our bodies' cells. Minerals also act as catalysts for biological functioning, digestion, muscle response, and hormone production.

One of the best examples of the effect of minerals on health comes from a people known as the Hunzas. Their water is so full of minerals, largely inorganic, that not only is it murky, but also the sediment settles at the bottom of the glass when it is allowed to stand. Yet these people have been known to have the best health of any people in the world.

Foods are often grown on exhausted, mineral-deficient soil and are then subjected to further depletion by refining and cooking. Moreover, as we grow older, the body's ability to absorb minerals decreases. Medications, illnesses, and poor eating habits further hamper proper absorption of minerals so that most of us suffer from at least some mineral deficiencies.

Enzymes

Enzymes are found in all living cells, including raw foods or those that are cooked at a temperature lower than 118 degrees Fahrenheit. Enzymes begin to perish when the temperature increases beyond this. The degree of enzyme destruction is a function of time and temperature.

Enzymes are needed to help control all mental and physical functions. They work with other substances such as minerals, vitamins, and proteins. Enzymes help extract the minerals from food, and they work with vitamins in every chemical reaction inside and outside the cells. Enzymes aid in transforming proteins into amino acids. Protein does not perform its function unless broken down into amino acids. Enzymes are responsible for nearly every facet of life and health and far outweigh the importance of every other nutrient.

Many experts believe that enzyme deficiency is a forerunner of disease and that nearly all people, because of improper diet over the years, need to replenish their enzyme supply. Enzymes are, therefore, justified as a supplemental dietary substance just as we add vitamins and minerals to our diet.

Vitamins

Vitamins are fascinating. They can give strength, and when properly directed, they can heal the oddest conditions the body can display. If we don't know enough about vitamins, it is due to our own neglect. We can't blame anyone else. We know and feel where our body is weak or aching, so we can do something about it.

Vitamins are not drugs! With enough minerals and a properly working digestive tract, the human body is able to manufacture vitamins all by itself. A properly functioning digestive tract makes all the B vitamins we need. The body can manufacture vitamins, but not minerals.

The following vitamins are manufactured by the body:

- The right collarbone manufactures vitamin A.
- The left collarbone manufactures vitamin B_{12}.
- The floating rib manufactures vitamin E.
- The healthy digestive system manufactures all of the B vitamins.
- The tailbone manufactures vitamin C.
- The red bone marrow manufactures vitamin K.
- The left leg manufactures linoleic acid.
- The small intestine manufactures interferon.
- The tip of the sternum is concerned with the right kind of vitamin D.

However, in this day and age when stress problems are prevalent, the miracle manufacturing plant in our body cannot function properly without outside help. Our needs are different from those of our ancestors.

We do not need as many calories as our hard-working ancestors needed. Their food was mostly homegrown, and contained no additives or preservatives. Nowadays, food stays preserved within our bodies longer. In the past, food did not undergo freezing processes, which remove vitamin E. There were no fluorescent lights, which rob vitamin A, and there was no pollution, which is known to rob vitamin C. Therefore, we need vitamins—*every one of us*. As you read the lists that follow, you can see how vitamins affect many parts of the body and associated conditions.

Vitamin A (carotene): Eyes, teeth, bones, hair, dry skin, pimples, soft tissues, nose, mouth, throat, tonsils, digestive tract, heartburn, male and female genital organs. Growth, allergies, colds, sinuses, bronchial tubes, kidney stones, gallstones. Take one milligram (mg.) per 50 pounds of body weight.

Vitamin C (ascorbic acid): Body cells, complexion, eyes, blood, arteries, veins, tissues, ligaments, bones, nails. Healing; resistance to shock; fights infection. Pyorrhea, bad teeth, allergies, diphtheria, influenza, dysentery, measles, mumps, shingles, fever blisters, chicken pox, polio, bruises, restlessness, irritability. Take 500 mg. daily.

Vitamin D: All glands; reproduction. Distributes calcium and phosphorus, makes skin breathe; activated by sunshine and energy. Lack of D causes rickets (soft bone disease), acne, arthritis, nearsightedness. Take 500 IU daily.

Vitamin E: Muscle tissue, nerves, liver, heart, circulation, pituitary glands, adrenal and sex glands, reproductive glands, hormone production. Life span, fertility/sterility, miscarriages, testicular degeneration, cerebral palsy, epilepsy, mental disorders, bursitis, rheumatism, ulcers, wounds, burns, varicose veins, softens scar tissue. Take 400 IU daily.

Vitamin K: Blood clotting. Take 100 mg. daily.

Vitamin B_1 (thiamine chloride): Nerves, heart, thyroid gland. Tiredness, stress, irritability, oversensitivity, memory, morale; appetite, nausea, constipation, digestion, metabolism of fats and carbohydrates. Take 25 mg. daily.

Vitamin B_2 (riboflavin): Skin, metabolism of starches and sugar, digestion, vision, longevity, reproduction, lactation. Athlete's foot, allergies. Take 25 mg. daily.

Niacin: Liver, nerves, soft tissues, skin, gums, digestion, circulation, burning of starches and sugars. Dual personality, cowardliness. Niacinamide is another name for niacin. Take 100 mg. daily.

Vitamin B_6 (pyridoxine): Muscle tone, nerves. Conserves protein. Acne, paralysis, dizziness, intolerance to sunshine, insomnia, fatigue, palsy, joint stiffness. Take 25 mg. daily.

Folate/folic acid: Red blood cells, anemia, poor appetite. Take 10 mg. daily.

Vitamin B$_{12}$ (cobalamin): Growth, blood. Pernicious anemia, nerve degeneration, asthma, skin disorders, fatigue, listlessness, paleness, unclear thinking. Take 500 micrograms (mcg.) daily.

Biotin: Mental health, muscles, dry skin, poor appetite, nausea, mental depression. Take 3 mg. daily.

Pantothenic acid: Growth, digestion, wrinkles, hair, adrenal glands, nerves. Stress, anemia, arthritis, constipation, stomach ulcers, water retention, edema. Take 100 mg. daily.

Choline: Metabolism of fats, liver, kidneys, spleen, gallbladder, nerves, muscles, skin; diabetes, arteriosclerosis (hardening of arteries), cancer, fatigue, gray hair. Valuable in all cases of dyspepsia and disorders of the stomach. Take 250 mg. daily.

Inositol: Liver, intestines, heart, muscles, nerves. Utilization of vitamins V and E, growth, brain functioning. Gray hair, hair loss. Take 250 mg. daily.

Rutin (bioflavonoids): Small blood vessels; high blood pressure, strokes, ankle swelling, allergies. Take 50 mg. daily.

Para-aminobenzoic acid (PABA): Thyroid gland, all other glands, hormone activation. Sterility, gray hair, arthritis. Take 100 mg. daily.

Vitamin F: Unsaturated fatty acids; lubricates all cells, skin, nails, hair. Lack of vitamin F causes bronchial asthma, hay fever, baldness, acne. Take 100 mg. daily.

Cell Salts (Tissue Salts)

In our search for truth, we have to consider one branch of food additives—the cell salt—found, invented, and documented by Dr. Schuessler 100 years ago. He found that by supplying the minimum dosage of 12 important minerals, the body responds extremely well.

Schuessler's tissue salts have a specific place in supplying the body and its cells with the needed building materials. Tissue salts, also called cell salts, are only vibrations of 12 fundamental minerals. But, being of vibrations *alone*, they nourish the finer body and rebuild the aura. They also stimulate and spark into action already-present minerals. Cell salts spark the entire metabolism by bringing together and catalyzing organic and inorganic mineral supplies.

There are twelve tissue salts:

1. **Calcium fluoride:** Deals with the treatment of ailments connected with bones, decaying teeth, blood, and relaxed conditions of muscle fibers such as falling womb, abortion, corpulence, and enlarged heart muscles.

2. **Calcium phosphate:** Noted for its effect on the skeletal frame of the body—heals delayed dentition, decaying teeth, bone deformities, and other skeletal affections. It is a valuable remedy for expectant mothers, especially for women who are incapable of carrying to full term. It has a sedative effect on the body, just like that of lime on the soil. It forms part of the blood corpuscles and gastric acid; therefore, it is effective in the treatment of anemia and gastritis.

3. **Calcium sulfate:** Known as a blood purifier and healer, it causes the discharge of decaying, organic matter. It is indicated for boils, ulcers, abscesses, and skin affections. It is normally used in conjunction with silica.

4. **Ferric phosphate** (iron): Known as the oxygen carrier, it could, therefore, be helpful in many illnesses. It is indicated in all inflammatory conditions and all cases characterized by a rise in temperature, such as fevers, colds, coughs, croup, bronchitis, pleurisy, measles, chicken pox, and pneumonia. It is also applicable in all anemia cases, iron being a constituent of the hemoglobin part of the red blood corpuscles.

5. **Kalium muriate** (potassium chloride): Indicated in cases of long-standing, sluggish conditions. Its symptoms are characterized by a white coating of the tongue, such as in diphtheria, croup, and pneumonia, and by thick white discharges affecting the skin and mucous membranes. It is useful when the blood tends to thicken and form clots.

6. **Kalium phosphate** (potassium phosphate): Associated with all nervous affections, such as nervous headaches and irritability; and, in fact, with all ailments originating from nervous tension, such as fretfulness, hysteria, and neuralgia. Children's tantrums could indicate a deficiency of this cell salt.

7. **Kalium sulfate** (potassium sulfate): An oxygen carrier; it is indicated when there is a feeling of stuffiness or a need for fresh air. It is noted for skin affections characterized by a yellow discharge, and it has been found helpful in maintaining healthy scalp and hair.

8. **Magnesium phosphate**: Indicated in cases characterized by spasmodic pains of the teeth, head, stomach, and abdomen. It helps in relieving muscular twitching and is noted for relieving nervous affections that produce convulsions, cramps, menstrual pains, and any other sharp twinges of pain. Flatulence can be relieved by this cell salt, making it a useful remedy for colic.

9. **Natrium muriate** (sodium chloride): Although this is common salt, it is capable of correcting cases that result from excessive use of common salt. Its indication is associated with body fluids and malnutrition, such as coryza, and it is known as the water-distributing tissue salt. A natrium muriate deficiency must be considered when there is excessive dryness or moisture in any part of the body or when an imbalance of the water system is indicated by, for example, eyes tearing, abnormal salivation, constipation, and so forth.

10. **Natrium phosphate** (sodium phosphate): Known as the acid neutralizer. It is useful in cases of worms, acidity, heartburn, and regurgitation—in fact, all gastric derangements. It has also been found helpful in cases of stiffness and swelling of joints.

11. **Natrium sulfate** (sodium sulfate): Indicated in all cases of biliousness, gallstones, nausea, and vomiting. It is known to eliminate excess water in the system that may contain toxic matter. It is essential to a healthy liver.

12. **Silica** (silicis oxide): A cleanser and eliminator noted for the relief of boils, ulcers, abscesses, and glandular swellings. In fact, it promotes

suppuration in all cases of tumors. Its action is rather sturdy, but deep-seated. It could effectively be used in alternation with calcium sulfate.

Exercise

Our bodies need exercise. The lymphatic system does not work without sufficient exercise. Protein assimilation depends on a properly working lymphatic system. So protein assimilation depends on exercise. Did you walk today? Try climbing your stairs an extra time tonight just for exercise—or use your trampoline a few minutes at a time.

Water

Water is an important component of the cells and tissues. It keeps tissues soft and pliable and acts as a solvent of gases and foods, permitting diffusion of these substances in the body. It is the medium of transport for food absorbed from the alimentary canal. Absorbed food is carried from the alimentary canal in the watery blood plasma to all parts of the body. Water enables glands to manufacture their particular secretions and assists in regulating body temperature. Harmful waste is carried in solution to excretory organs.

The body consists of 90 percent water. Water is the most important "food" intake. Fluid is needed for assimilation and transmutation of minerals and vitamins. Foods and oxygen cannot be used without fluids. Therefore, I urge you to drink healthful fluids, such as fresh juices, good water, herbal teas, and buttermilk, instead of liquor, alcohol, soda pop, and junk drinks.

To make positive vion-rich water (vions are ions of the water), take a jar of water and place it between two horseshoe magnets. The positive and negative poles of the magnets should be facing each other, causing them to repel each other.

Sunshine, Negative Ions, and Full-Spectrum Lighting

For the past 50 years, our society has lived and worked more and more inside. No one has ever calculated the side effects of this behavior as a whole. All of us are lacking sunshine and the negative ions that nature provides so freely.

What about bringing these into our homes? We know about the healthful effects of negative ions. Sleep is deeper and more restful. We are more alert at work. We live happier lives. Airborne allergies vanish. Asthma is lessened. Behavior-troubled children are calmed down and sleep a restful night.

The trouble with us is that we hear of negative ions and we think that more is better. We need to realize that while we can read comfortably with a 75-watt reading lamp, we cannot read when we put 10,000 watts in the lamp. So it is with negative ions. If we overcharge the room, the body cannot absorb or utilize the unnatural balance of negative ions.

We all agree that we do not have enough sunlight in our homes. Full-spectrum lighting fixtures (a combination of black light with chroma light) truly are remarkable. It is sunshine indoors. When we combine full-spectrum lighting with negative ions, we bring the outdoors inside.

The following results of concrete studies illustrate the advantages of full-spectrum lighting:

- Hyperactivity was greatly lessened in schoolchildren under these lights.
- Eyestrain was eliminated.
- Fewer cavities were noted.
- Fewer colds were noted.
- Greater muscle strength was noted.
- Reduction of airborne bacteria was noted.
- Greater visual acuity with less illumination was noted.

Full-spectrum lighting cures certain types of depression, combats fatigue, increases work capacity, reduces high blood pressure, reduces the amount of insulin needed by diabetics, tends to restore hormonal balance, strengthens the body's immune system, quickens the healing process—especially of bones—and the list goes on.

Without the light of the sun with its varied wavelengths (x-ray, ultraviolet, infrared, visible, radio, etc.), life as we know it could not exist. Light is and was that which forms the blueprint for the evolving forms of life on this planet. As our earth's atmosphere filters the sun's rays, it provides only a specific aggregate of light wavelengths to reach the surface. As life evolved on this sphere, it did so under a very specific combination of wavelengths, the quality of which had the effect of enhancing or inhibiting the evolution of specific life forms. That which we see around us today and call *life* is the direct effect of sunlight over eons, playing upon the environment of our planet.

The need for sunlight is much the same as our need for food, and, just as one either nourishes or starves the body through one's dietary intake of food, so it is with light. Humans are attuned both physiologically and psychologically to the subtle energies of light. Since the beginning of time, light has tuned the strings of our bodies to play a multitude of symphonies, which we call *life processes*.

We need only look to the agricultural industry to see the effect of a change in the natural environment on the life processes of living things. It has been cost-effective and more efficient to raise animals in a closed environment, but in doing so we have incurred a multitude of challenges. Feeds must be fortified to assure that some (hopefully enough) of the nutrients reach the vital areas of the body in order to maintain adequate health—yet disease flourishes. Multiple vaccinations against diseases that are unheard of in a natural environment have become a must. Overall performance of the animals has been drastically reduced by keeping them in a closed environment.

Full-spectrum lighting is an artificial lighting system that re-creates a natural outdoor light environment at an intensity level that is safe. The concept of a system must be emphasized here because there are lights on the market today that claim to be "full-spectrum" but that, in the true definition of the concept, are not. These other lights either do not provide a full spectrum for the length of the life of the bulb, or they produce more than a full spectrum of light, such as the production of x-rays or radiation in the form of radio frequencies, which have been shown to cause, among other things, a gross loss of muscles strength.

Unlike animals that have been forced into living in closed environments to suit *our* purposes, we *chose* long ago to live that way. Yet we, like the animals, inherit the difficulties that arise from separating ourselves from the natural light environment under which we evolved.

Even glass—which allows visible light to brighten enclosed space—blocks out part of the natural spectrum of sunlight. Dr. Richard Wurtman, the world-renowned neuroendocrinologist, has pioneered contemporary research on the effects of light on living things and has traced visual pathways in humans, which are independent of the optic tract. These lead to brain centers that control, among other things, endocrine function and metabolic activity. These photoreceptors (or light-sensitive receptors) in the eye respond to specific wavelengths of light found in natural sunlight, and they serve to regulate and reinforce normal functioning of bodily processes. In other words, the composite spectrum of normal sunlight acts as a computer card to the brain via the photoreceptors in the eyes, reinforcing and stabilizing the harmony in bodily processes that have evolved over countless ages under the full-spectrum influence of the sun. Many natural wavelengths of radiant energy found in sunlight that reach the surface of our planet are not even present in artificial light sources. It may be said that all artificial light sources emit a distorted sun spectrum or emit additional frequencies not found in sunlight. This results in overstimulation, understimulation, or no stimulation at all to the photoreceptors in the eyes.

For those who must wear corrective eye lenses, there is a special plastic lens available that allows the full spectrum of sunlight to penetrate the eye.

Most assuredly, our bodies are miraculous in their ability to adapt and recuperate under unfavorable circumstances. Yet, such is the steady pressure of this seemingly subtle influence of light that, after repeated and prolonged exposure to artificial lighting, our brain centers succumb to these distorted signals, and things begin to go awry.

Full-spectrum lighting, which grounds radio frequencies emitted by fluorescent lights and shields cathodes, has never shown any type of harmful effect on any living thing that evolved under the spectrum of sunlight. This is definitely not the case with conventional fluorescent tubes, high intensity discharge lamps, or metal halide lamps.

Kinesiology

We are affected by everything in our environment, either positively or negatively. One of the ways that we can determine which things affect us positively and which negatively is through muscle testing.

Use the following procedure to test for positive and negative muscle reactions.

1. Have the subject stand erect, left arm relaxed at the side, right arm held out parallel to the floor, with elbow straight.

2. Face the subject and place your left hand on the subject's extended right arm just above the wrist.

3. Tell the subject you are going to try to push his arm down as he resists with all his strength.

4. Now push down on his arm quickly and firmly. The idea is to push just hard enough to test the spring and bounce in the arm, but not so hard that the muscle becomes fatigued. It is not a question of who is stronger, but of whether the muscle can lock the shoulder joint against the push.

5. Now put the item to be tested in your subject's left hand and check again.

    —   If the food or item is good for the subject, the arm will lock in place and stay strong.

    —   If the item is not good for the subject, you will be able to push the arm down. Any food or item that muscle-tests weakly is not good for the subject. You could say that it weakens him or that the subject is allergic to it.

Test all foods you eat. This technique is also good for vitamin and herb testing. Remember that one vitamin may test positive, but when you take a bunch of different vitamins at the same time, they may weaken you. Put all the vitamins in your left hand and test whether they can be taken together.

Dr. Emanuel Cheraskin of the University of Alabama Dental School has authored 13 books on the relationship between diet and disease. His work included studies on what we eat and how it affects us.

"Americans have the worst diet in the world," Cheraskin tells us. "And even doctors, who should know better, are not eating enough of the right foods to keep them healthy."

But the worst offenders are teenage girls. "Teen-age boys eat a little better and get more nutrition, simply because they eat more than girls do," he explains. "People in their 30s and 40s also are busy building physical deficiencies that are bound to result in serious illnesses later.

"There is evidence now to indicate that poor eating habits might be responsible for many more types of illnesses than science ever imagined," claims Cheraskin. "Even infertility, mental retardation, heart disease, and cancer may be directly related to poor nutrition."

It looks like we are what we eat after all. And what we eat is usually a lot of garbage. So, if we don't do something about our diet, we may all wind up in serious trouble.

But there is hope. Some of the people who took part in Cheraskin's studies and who had damaged their health by poor eating habits have turned their health around through a proper diet.

Mental Attitude Is Your Responsibility

Neglect in the mental realm can cause trouble in the physical body. Inform yourself by reading or listening to ideas and alternatives; this helps to remedy the specializations we endure in our society nowadays.

Read a little every day or listen to worthwhile tapes while you drive or wash your dishes. It is said that we use only 10 percent of our brain capacities. If we do not exercise the brain, its potential drops.

Your Spiritual Responsibility:
Do Not Neglect Prayer, Meditation, and Contemplation!

Have you said your morning prayers? Did you protect your aura? Every culture and every civilization has had—or has—a method of protecting the human aura from foreign, undesirable influences.

The American Indians raised their arms and asked their spirits for protection—not only for themselves, but also for the animal and plant kingdoms. The Japanese use candles and perform candle ceremonies. The Christians hold the cross or the Bible and ask Jesus for the light and its protection.

All cultures realize that neglecting the spiritual body can cause difficulties in the course of the day. In any case, I recommend strongly that you not neglect your spiritual body. Nourishing it only once a week on Sunday morning in church is not enough.

It is true that honest prayer makes a blue light. A blue light is a power, an energy that is of a creative nature. Bless your food, and the blue light of your blessing will make your food a healing food. Bless your water, and it will become a healing water. Bless your child and pray over your beloved ones, and the blue light will heal the fluid that will reach the very cells, and the cells will obey the light.

Cause and Effect

Cause is in consciousness—the unseen.
Effect is in circumstances—the seen.

When the effect is in circumstances involving health, you can be sure that your consciousness is causing this. But how? The key is in negativity.

What follows are ten major areas where negativity may enter consciousness. Convert this negativity to positivity—this will create a consciousness of continued good health.

TEN COMMANDMENTS FOR MAINTAINING PERFECT HEALTH

1. *Accept criticism as the other person's problem, not yours.*

2. *Appreciate yourself and reaffirm your self-worth whenever necessary.*

3. *See the good points in circumstances. See even problems as happening for the best.*

4. *Rather than looking backward with sorrow, look forward with joyous expectation.*

5. *Rather than fretting about what you do not have, appreciate what you have.*

6. *Learn from mistakes so that you can convert them into triumphs.*

7. *Insulate yourself from distasteful surroundings through wholesome detachment.*

8. *Let go of what you no longer need, and make the most of what you now attract.*

9. *Grow in courage and self-mastery from every circumstance.*

10. *Be aware of the larger consciousness of which you are a part.*

These might be called the ten commandments for good health. They are beyond the physical—in the unseen world of consciousness. Observe them and enjoy perfect health.

❧ CHAPTER TWO ❧

Trauma As a Cause of Ill Health

Trauma comes not only from accidental injuries, but from operations as well. An injury rocks the aura; an operation cuts the aura. An injury offsets the aura; an operation makes holes in the aura. In either case, an aura has to be mended after it is hurt.

Shock will injure the aura. In all cases of injuries, there are two things to be done: Heal the injured part, and heal the aura. In my opinion, healing the aura is almost more important, as the following story illustrates.

Mrs. Worthington was a good customer in my little store. We talked about many spiritual things. When she entered my establishment, I pushed all work aside just to chat with her. She used to study with the Kahunas and the masters of Easter Island, and she nourished my curious mind.

One day we heard a terrible scream outside. We both rushed to see what it was. A woman lay on the sidewalk. Obviously, she had slipped. The bone of her right leg was sticking out of the skin—broken, blood oozing. We helped her into a more comfortable position. Then I ran to call the ambulance. Looking back, I saw Mrs. Worthington kneel in front of the leg. Using her big, massive body to shield what she was doing from the spectators, she swished her hands over the leg, back and forth, and murmured some kind of secret formula. I was slow in finding the number of the ambulance. I could not get through quickly enough; it took much longer than it should have. When I got back outside, my friend was still murmuring, bent over the woman's leg, but there was no longer any skin broken and no bone sticking out. A peaceful look on the face of the injured woman showed that there was no longer any pain either.

I still thank God that the ambulance took so long and I could see the miracle happen before my eyes. The bone looked straight now, no swelling. The wound was closed, and Mrs. Worthington urged the patient to move her feet. When the ambulance finally arrived, we helped the woman up. She stood on both feet saying thank you to us. Later on, I heard that she went home the next day because there was no more trouble.

I pulled Mrs. Worthington into the shop. "Please tell me what you did. Tell me how you did it."

"Oh, not much," this humble woman said. "I just mended the aura of the bone, and there was time enough for the bone to heal itself."

"Where did you learn this?" I asked.

"It is the teaching of the sages on Easter Island that I applied here. I really don't know much. I just learned to heal bones, that's all," she said.

This experience gave me an insight into healing—a lesson I will never forget.

Osteopathic Medicine

In a small town in Kansas a century ago, a country physician announced that he had abandoned orthodox medicine in order to found his own healing system. He persisted in this course despite fierce opposition from the medical profession. He gained a devoted following and, thus, launched osteopathy. Dr. Andrew Taylor Still was a colorful physician who grew up in the traditions of frontier medicine. His father, Dr. Abram Still, was a Methodist medical missionary serving Indian tribes.

Dr. Andrew Still was born on August 6, 1828, in Jonesboro, Virginia. He learned medicine from his father and later attended courses at the Kansas City College of Physicians and Surgeons. It has been said that as a young man he roamed the prairies, digging up graves so that he could learn anatomy by dissecting corpses.

He served as a militia officer and hospital steward in the Civil War, then settled in Baldwin, Kansas. When three of his children died of spinal meningitis, he turned against the medical practices of the day—especially the use of massive medications—and began to devise his own system. He became convinced that spinal dislocation was a root cause of illness, creating pressures on nerves and blood vessels that either led to a direct breakdown, or else so weakened the body that it lost its natural resistance to disease.

Herbs and Trauma

There are some dependable herbs for trauma conditions. Arnica Montana has many names, such as mountain daisy, leopard's bane, and mountain tobacco. Arnica has bright chrome-yellow flowers. The plant can reach a height of nearly two feet. You can use it topically—make a strong tea, then take a soft towel, soak it in the warm tea, and apply it over bruises, dislocations, corns, bunions, carbuncles, boils, and insect bites. Arnica is beneficial in all injuries when they are *not open sores or broken skin.*

For inner bruises, take arnica as a tincture or in homeopathic form. When a person has had prenatal injuries—an arm too short or fingers undeveloped—try arnica in high dosage and see miracles happen.

Another flower that acts quickly is the common daisy. When you perform unaccustomed work, such as lawn mowing, gardening, mountain climbing, or too much roller skating, and muscles become stiff, turn to our lovely daisy. Make a brew of daisies and, again, use a soft towel to apply it to your sore muscles. Also, several spoonfuls of daisy tea taken orally are very helpful to stiff and sore muscles. You may want to keep daisy tincture in your cupboard just to have it ready.

The Biblical herb *rue* is a very special one. For painfully twisted wrists or elbows, or for overworked tendons, make a concoction with rue and apply it to the painful arm. In only a few days, the wrist will be normal again. Rue works on the upper part of the body. As an eyesight restorer, it is the most incredible herb, giving the "Ray of Light" back to the aging eye. Make rue tea using one teaspoon rue to one cup of water and steep five minutes. Drink one cup two times daily.

St. John's wort (*Hypericum perforatum*) also belongs in the "trauma medicine chest." It can accomplish many things, such as:

- closing the lips of a wound.
- relieving pain, particularly toothaches.
- dissolving swelling.
- opening obstructions.
- repairing nerve damage.

Acupressure and Contact Healing

One of the most outstanding inventors on this earth today is Rev. Dr. Fred Houston. He is the man who found an acupressure method that works for Westerners. His tremendous book on contact healing should be in every house. It is called *The Healing Benefits of Acupressure*.

He gave me permission to demonstrate how to get rid of old traumatic conditions. Stand in front of the friend who needs help. Slide your hands over his shoulder and hold the notch where the scapula attaches to the arm joint. Feel around a little, and if the area is sore, hold it. Let your friend close his eyes and experience what happens. Sometimes an old operation site starts burning or gets warm, or a bone starts hurting or gets warm. Hold it until all sensations are gone (between five and ten minutes). That is enough for one day. If needed, repeat the next day until there is no more pain or warm areas evident.

This is a terrific method for getting rid of old injuries.

Foot Reflex Massage

Foot reflex massage is a scientific massage of the feet that can be performed without using any mechanical devices. Only the hands of the therapist do the work, and the healing forces can work directly. But this massage does not serve only the feet and legs—it treats the whole human being. There are exactly localized reflex zones in all parts of the body. The treatment of these reflexes often works so well that it is without a doubt superior to any other kind of treatment. Thousands of years ago, people of high culture knew about this treatment.

Every human being has reflexes in the feet, but they are only painful if the related organ is overstrained, weakened, affected, or really sick. This method gives the therapist a pretty good picture of what should be treated.

Foot reflexology can prevent long suffering. It is important to know about the reactions. They are desirable, and they are a sign that a person still has enough strength to heal himself and get rid of toxins. The reactions are individually very different. Some are disagreeable, but they do not last too long and do help to reestablish health.

The most common reactions are as follows:

- Relaxation and deeper sleep
- Secretion of more urine (cleaning blood and kidneys)
- Changes in the urine, causing it to be turbid and darker
- More bowel movements
- Secretions from nose and throat

Foot reflexology plays an important part in traumatic and congestive disorders.

Simple Technique for Hiccups

Dr. Joseph Stapczynski, an emergency medicine specialist, advises, "Take an ear swab and gently massage the back area of the roof of your mouth where it is soft and fleshy for approximately one minute. If you are unsure of where this fleshy roof area begins, you can gently run your finger back along the roof of your mouth until you feel where the hard area ends and the soft area begins."

This remarkably effective technique works by actually interrupting the hiccup reflex, doctors believe. It has worked on 100 percent of patients.

Circulation

Try this method to stimulate circulation: First, hold the area in front of the ears, on both sides, for about one minute. Then, using the right hand an inch or so away from the body, make ten clockwise circles over the heart. Then, do the same thing over the thymus.

Bones

Our bones are very sensitive to street drugs. Years after someone has taken LSD and other similar drugs, the bones are—and stay—weakened. A small fall or a wrong step and a bone breaks. When I find someone with weak bones who is not a senior citizen, I know that the body was abused with drugs.

To know if your bones are broken or weak, touch the seventh vertebra. If it is sore, your bones cry out for help. (This is Dr. Fred Houston's method.)

Bonemeal, calcium orotate, vitamin C, comfrey root, oat straw tea, and an oat straw mattress are all bone strengthening.

~≪ CHAPTER THREE ≫~

Congestion As a Cause of Ill Health

Congestion needs short fasts and herbs. Just as a surgeon and physician use different instruments for different procedures, so can we use different fasts and different herbal teas to accomplish this cleaning out.

Have you ever been in debt? If so, you know how difficult it is to pay debts off. You have to work three times as hard, first to make a living, second to pay back the debts, and third to pay back the interest. It is the same with your body. Debts of negligence to your body cannot be repaid with one injection or by skipping alcohol for a day or two.

Using an injection or a pill to be free from pain will not heal your body. Whoever lives against the laws of nature is losing valuable and happy years. Whoever lives within the laws of nature is on the winning side, gaining happy, healthy years.

Arteriosclerosis and Atherosclerosis

Arteriosclerosis is a term applied to a pathological condition in which the walls of blood vessels, especially the arteries, experience thickening, hardening, and loss of elasticity. In short, it is the hardening of the arteries. Atherosclerosis takes place when arteries are blocked and the blood cannot pass through freely.

Long before a stroke and/or heart attack comes to pass, there is buildup in the arteries. It builds up over the years. Arteriosclerosis is no longer a disease of senior citizens, but also of men in their 30s and younger. Recently, researchers found arterial changes in infants. Even women, who were thought to have immunity to arteriosclerosis, suffer more and more from this disease.

When physicians speak of arteriosclerosis, they compare the disease with the plague of the Middle Ages. The question is: Why are so many people plagued with the buildup of junk in their arteries? Arteriosclerosis and atherosclerosis are two sides of the same coin. The first one is the hardening of the elastic tubes—the arteries—and the filling up of these tubes with sludge and blood corpuscles. The second one occurs when fat deposits in and around the arteries choke the passage of blood and bring on complete stoppage. The final result of both is heart attack or stroke.

Herbal Chelation

Herbs, vitamins, minerals, and amino acids are a godsend for our health. We can help ourselves by using these important supplements to attain excellent health. They can do wonders for the heart and circulation.

Doctors in Germany recommend hawthorn for people with heart disease. They have learned and applied what herbalists have known for hundreds of years—that hawthorn helps the heart. It is wonderful for problems associated with atherosclerosis, high blood pressure, and elevated cholesterol levels. Hawthorn also strengthens heart contractions, lowering blood pressure and pulse rate.

Equisetum arvense is the Latin term for horsetail, which one French medical journal described as having healing properties for the heart. *Equisetum* contains elemental silicon, which is necessary for maintaining flexible arterial walls. As we get older, we have less and less silicon and must take *Equisetum* to make up for this loss. When *Equisetum* is combined with hawthorn, the results are amazing. *Equisetum* acts like a broom for the arteries and increases the number of blood corpuscles.

People with heart disease lack chromium and selenium. Our food used to supply us with these minerals, but now the soil is losing precious nutrients due to overfarming and harsh chemical fertilizers. Animals who graze on selenium-depleted soils have weakened heart muscles. Chromium is very important because it improves the ratio of "good" cholesterol to "bad" cholesterol and keeps the overall cholesterol level down. We should consider supplementing with these minerals to avoid complications.

Amino acids can be remarkable for the heart, especially taurine and arginine. Taurine is known to help with hardening of the arteries, high blood pressure, and even congestive heart failure. This amino acid protects against potassium depletion of the heart, which can lead to seriously irregular heartbeats. Taurine is needed to maintain proper blood platelet functioning. The amino acid arginine is the only source for nitric oxide, which is vital to relax the arterial walls so that blood can flow more freely, resulting in more healthy blood vessels.

Vitamin C helps with blood clotting and high cholesterol levels. It also maintains capillary wall strength. Vitamin C and selenium are important antioxidants for those with heart conditions, since they protect against stroke.

What to Do

The ingredients discussed above are so divine that they have been referred to as Our Lord's Formula. Aloe vera gel is also recommended to keep circulation flowing. Take this *Herbal Chelation* formula—a combination of hawthorn berries, *Equisetum* concentrate, vitamin C, taurine, arginine, chromium picolinate, and selenium—with two tablespoons aloe vera gel before each meal three times daily. You can take aloe vera gel alone or put it in apple juice or water, but *not* in citrus juices. Do this for one month and then have your physician recheck the health of your arteries. If it is not all gone, repeat. Do not eat heavy meals, potato chips, heavy cakes, alcohol, or strong coffee.

In order to keep arteries clear afterwards, consider the French method: Take one kelp tablet and one choline tablet (250 mg.) two times daily.

Yogurt and applesauce also help keep arteries clean.

Symptoms of Arteriosclerosis

The following symptoms are likely to appear in your body when plaque is building up in the arteries.

- Overly tired feeling after a heavy meal
- Forgetfulness with tasks that you normally perform with acuity
- Inability to grasp new ideas or follow new dimensions

- Persistent feelings of weakness, coldness, and tingling or burning in your toes or feet
- Dull headaches
- Persistent sleeplessness
- Tightness in chest
- Pain in shoulders—if not accident related
- Breathlessness when walking or lifting
- Pain in the calves of the legs caused by walking (when you rest, you feel better, and pain disappears)
- Sharp pain in the middle of the sternum when stretching or exercising (it goes away but returns the next morning)
- Small ulcerations of the skin on ankles or feet
- Head noises, dizziness, sudden spells of partial deafness
- Blurred or darkened vision

Symptoms of Advanced Arteriosclerosis

The first signs of plaque buildup in the arteries are not easily recognized, as already discussed. If a person is stricken by advanced arteriosclerosis, symptoms include having to make very small steps and having to rest every 100 to 200 yards because of pain in feet and/or legs, particularly calves. Sometimes the person limps (called claudication), but this is always accompanied by pain. That can be arteriosclerosis in the lower extremities.

The following illnesses may have, as an underlying cause, blockage in the arteries—a plaque buildup in the arteries so that blood and oxygen are not sufficiently supplied to the different organs of the body:

- Asthma
- High blood pressure
- Loss of sleep
- Loss of eyesight
- Lymph trouble
- Kidney trouble
- Prostate trouble
- Heart trouble
- Loss of memory
- Loss of hearing
- Leg pain
- Liver trouble
- Diabetes
- Stroke

It sounds harsh, but there is no better prevention and correction of the above disease patterns than the cleaning of your arteries.

When diseased, the venous system also can make pain and give trouble similar to arterial blockage. Here is the difference to observe: With an arterial blockage, walking briskly causes tightness and pain to start in the calves and feet, but this lets up when you stand for a little while. With venous system blockage, pain diminishes as you walk, but when you stand still, pain increases.

Causes of Arteriosclerosis and Atherosclerosis

Experts tell us that the causes of arteriosclerosis and atherosclerosis include the following:

- Too much fat intake
- Too many chemicals in water, food, and air
- Too many metal poisons in water, food, and air
- Too much sodium fluoride buildup
- Too much sugar (more than six teaspoons at one time causes blood to coagulate, making tiny blood clots)
- Too much environmental stress
- Too little exercise
- Too much smoking
- Birth-control pills
- Noise pollution

Kurt Oster, M.D., tells us that milk, if not soured as in yogurt or kefir, cannot be utilized totally. His xanthine oxidase theory sounds promising and would seem to be borne out by the following case.

In 1945, a hospital in Milwaukee designed for mentally disturbed senior citizens was supervised by E. Seiler, M.D., a psychiatrist. She ordered all milk removed from the diet. Only yogurt was permitted once a day. Patients had plenty of butter, oils, vegetables, eggs, and meats, but no milk or ice cream. The result was astounding. After three months, the patients became rational and could be taken home. Many of them remained well for years.

Test Your Own Arterial Health

Try the following methods to test your own arterial health.

Foot Test—Walk barefoot for two minutes outside, in the grass if possible. Then lie on your back and stretch your legs upwards. Ask someone to look at the soles of your feet. If they show white spots, it indicates that your leg arteries are narrowed down, and not enough blood can reach your foot.

Fist Test—take these steps:

1. Lift both hands above your head.
2. Make fists with firm pressure.
3. Open and close fists ten times.
4. Ask someone to hold your wrists firmly.
5. Open and close again ten times.
6. Your helper should release the grip on your wrists quickly. In four seconds your hands should be really red. If not, you have arterial trouble in your upper torso.

Eye Test—Look in the mirror. Around the colored part of the eye you will find a white ring.

Ear Test—Look at your earlobes. A crease in the left earlobe or a star of wrinkles shows arterial trouble around the heart.

Where Is the Blockage?

You can find out where the blockage is located by noting the following symptoms:

- Pain around hips, and the muscle you sit on becoming lame easily, may indicate plaque buildup in the aorta.
- Pain in the thigh may indicate sclerotic buildup in the midsection.
- Pain in the calves may indicate arterial trouble in arteries leading to legs.

- Pain in the feet and toes may indicate a plaque buildup of arteries supplying blood to the feet.

Seneca Indian Cleansing Diet

This diet was contributed by the Seneca Indians.

First day—Eat only fruits and all you want. Try apples, berries, watermelon, pears, peaches, cherries, whole citrus fruits, and so forth. No bananas.

Second day—Drink all the herbal teas you want, such as raspberry, hyssop, chamomile, or peppermint. You may sweeten the tea slightly with honey or maple sugar.

Third day—Eat all the vegetables you want. Have them raw, steamed, or both.

Fourth day—Make a big pot of vegetable broth by boiling cauliflower, cabbage, onion, green pepper, parsley, or whatever you have available. Season with sea salt or vegetable broth cubes. Drink only this rich mineral broth all day long.

This diet has the following effect: On the first day, you cleanse the colon (your wastebasket). On the second day, you release toxins, salt, and excessive calcium deposits in the muscles, tissues, and organs. On the third day, the digestive tract is supplied with healthful, mineral-rich bulk. On the fourth day, the blood, lymph, and inner organs are mineralized. That makes a lot of sense!

Aloe Vera Gel Cleanses Your Arteries

What is aloe vera? Aloe vera is a plant that has been used for medicinal purposes for centuries. It has been known for its therapeutic advantages and healing properties for more than 4,000 years. Ancient and modern literature abounds with references to this unique, natural vegetable remedy. It is sometimes called the medicine, miracle, or burn plant; it has many other names.

As early as 333 B.C., the Greeks identified aloe vera as a medicinal herb. The Chinese considered aloe vera sacred and used it for stomach and colon ailments. In the Philippines, it is used with milk for dysentery and kidney infections. Egyptians used it for sunburns and to retard the aging process.

Aloe vera aids in assimilation, circulation, and elimination. It has been reported to increase endurance and energy and to provide a speedy recovery from fatigue. It has been known to aid in muscle function and the utilization of vitamins and minerals. Aloe vera assists in achieving healthy skin and hair.

Aloe vera gel is not a drug. It does not react with medications.

Some of aloe vera's ingredients are listed below.

Active Ingredients	Minerals	Vitamins
Amino acids	Calcium	A
Enzymes	Magnesium	E
Natal aloes	Sodium	K
Aloin	Potassium	B_1
Emodin	Strontium	B_2
Bitter resins	Boron	B_3
Barbaloin	Silicon	B_6
Chlorophyll	Copper	Folic Acid
Albumin	Manganese	Choline
Essential oils	Iron	
Gum arabic	Aluminum	
Silica	Lithium	
Phosphate of zinc	Nickel	
	Zinc	

Aloe vera also provides the following benefits:

- Pain killer
- Fungicidal
- Germicidal
- Virucidal
- Anti-inflammatory (similar to steroid effects)
- Antipyretic (reduces fever and heat of sores)
- Natural cleanser

- Penetrates tissue
- Dilates capillaries
- Enhances normal cell proliferation (regenerative stage of healing)
- Reduces bleeding time

Cholesterol

As already mentioned, arteriosclerosis and atherosclerosis are two sides of the same coin. With atherosclerosis, a fatty, waxy substance clogs arteries inside and out. The Greek word *athere* means "porridge" or "gruel," and atherosclerosis is the buildup in the blood vessels of a gruel-like substance called cholesterol. "The arteries are so plugged up in some autopsy subjects, that no blood can get through at all," commented a first-year medical student.

This abnormal condition with its fatal consequences has caused more controversy over the last ten years than the bubonic plague, and it has been called the plague of modern times. It causes 55 percent of all deaths in the United States and has been the leading cause of death in our country since 1920. Scientists estimate that everyone over the age of 21 suffers to some extent from atherosclerosis and/or arteriosclerosis.

Because of the epidemic proportions this disease has reached, 20 percent of all research monies spent are used to study it, and some interesting findings are being disclosed. Cholesterol is absolutely essential to the body for the production of bile, for fat absorption in the intestines, for steroid hormone synthesis, and as an element in cell membranes. Why do we have trouble with cholesterol buildup when the body needs cholesterol? Atherosclerosis is a complex biochemical problem with no simple answers.

The liver is supposed to make the right amount of cholesterol. A poor liver being overworked and maltreated makes shortcuts so that the cholesterol amount is larger and more like glue.

The Truth about Cholesterol

Eskimos are on a high-fat, high-protein diet. They show very high cholesterol, but no arteriosclerosis is found. Their arteries are free of cholesterol buildup. Why?

Cholesterol has two chemicals. LDL, which stands for low-density lipoprotein, brings the cholesterol from the liver to the tissue. HDL, which stands for high-density lipoprotein, removes the excess cholesterol from tissues and arteries. It cleanses the arteries—I call it the "Ajax of the arteries."

Eskimos have lots of HDL; therefore, their arteries are clean in spite of the high consumption of fats and proteins. By the way, Eskimos also have very efficient kidneys to handle all the protein they consume.

A Japanese laboratory found that a special hormone is formed in the right shinbone that is picked up by the white corpuscles and delivered to the liver to be used for cholesterol processing. In some cases, this hormone is in short supply, and cholesterol-triglyceride trouble starts.

Here is an herbal combination that helps create the missing hormone: Okra, male fern, beth root, rhubarb root, and calamus root.

A cup of tea made from arnica and hyssop three times daily is also helpful.

What to Do

There are a number of things we can do to help keep our bodies free of cholesterol buildup.

- Stop smoking. Nicotine constricts arteries, so less blood can circulate through the constricted vessels.
- Walk more, and get more weight-bearing exercise.
- Use garlic to make arteries soft and pliable.
- B-complex helps a lot.
- Avoid noise pollution; it weakens the arteries. Workers subjected to loud music or working under motor noises are prone to high blood pressure.
- Avoid too much salt.
- Avoid too much sugar.
- Use choline; it relaxes the arteries, and helps in the fibrillation and irregularity of the heartbeat. Choline is easily counteracted by the enzyme cholinesterase; therefore, it has to be taken frequently. In its natural form, it is better accepted, and there is an abundance of cho-

line in wheat germ, malt, and grapes. If you combine choline tablets with kelp tablets, cholinesterase cannot counteract choline so easily.

- Use bee pollen as a terrific food supplement—one-quarter teaspoon two times daily will do.
- Use folic acid to build the "Ajax of the arteries"—HDL.
- Clean out your arteries with *Herbal Chelation* and aloe vera gel.

Protect Your Arteries

It is important for you to keep your arteries clean. What follows is a simple method that comes from England. It is highly recommended as a once-a-year treatment to protect your arteries.

First day—Grind up one almond, place in one cup of water, and drink.

Second day—Take two almonds, place in one cup of water, and drink.

Third day, etc.—Take three almonds, and so on until you have reached fifteen almonds. Then go down step by step until you are back to one almond a day. This also is the best remedy I know to prevent cancer.

Decongest Your Body

Once there is a buildup of toxins in the body, you need to get rid of them to maintain your health. Use the following methods to decongest your body.

Decongest Your Blood

Your blood and platelets form an unwanted gluelike substance. If gluelike substances in the blood are allowed to accumulate, the platelets release a dangerous waste called adenosine diphosphate (ADP). Once ADP is released, other platelets glue together. They form clumps that obstruct the flow of blood through the vessel, and this may lead to blood clots in the heart (heart attack), in the brain (stroke), in the lungs, or in any other vital organ.

To counteract this, take some onions and cut them into pieces. Add to water and simmer to make onion water. White and red onions together have more anticlotting power. Drink one-half cup onion water five times daily and take 50 mg. of B_6 with each one-half cup of onion water. Bananas and tomatoes, rice and millet are allowed. Do this for two days in a row. Then begin a good healthy diet, but continue with vitamin B_6. Red clover leaf tea is excellent, also.

You are as old as your arteries. Old age sets in when arteries are blocked. Old age sets in when parts of your body do not receive enough oxygen or nourishment due to diminished blood supply. My advice: Clean your arteries with *Herbal Chelation* and aloe vera gel.

Decongest Your Bronchial Tubes, Sinuses, and Lungs

Accumulated gluelike sludge can be loosened and eliminated with the following one- or two-day diet: Take a glass of warm water, squeeze the juice of one-half to one lemon into it, add a little honey, and drink this slowly. Make yourself lots of these drinks throughout the day, about ten glasses, one every hour or so.

This will decongest your bronchi, sinuses, and lungs. If needed, repeat it every week until all is clear. Do not eat any dry food with it.

Cleanse Your Body with a Lemon Cocktail

Use the following recipe to make a lemon drink that will clean out your system.

Combine: Juice of one-half lemon with one glass of medium hot or cold water. For each glass, add one or two tablespoons of pure maple syrup, or use sorghum or natural molasses that does not contain sulfur dioxide.

How to use: Take from 8 to 20 glasses of the cocktail every 24 hours. If at any time you become weak or nervous, you may have a glass of strained orange juice during the day, but take no other food during the fast.

To break the fast: One glass of unstrained orange juice may be taken for breakfast in place of the cocktail. A serious mistake is often made when too much food is taken after a fast, and injury to the system is the result. Only light, nourishing food should be taken during the first two days after the fast.

For those who are overweight, less syrup or molasses may be taken, and only about six to eight glasses of the cocktail. An enema, night and morning, is recommended by most doctors for elimination. A cup of laxative herbal tea may be taken at bedtime if needed. One teaspoon of slippery elm taken with the cocktail two or three times during the day is recommended for an irritated stomach.

Lemon is a loosening and cleansing agent. Its 49 percent potassium level strengthens and energizes the heart, its oxygen builds vitality, its carbon acts as a motor stimulant, its hydrogen activates the sensory nervous system, its calcium strengthens and builds the lungs, its phosphorus knits the bones, its sodium encourages tissue building, its magnesium acts as a blood alkalizer, its iron builds red corpuscles, its chlorine cleanses the blood plasma, and its silicon aids the thyroid for deeper breathing.

The maple syrup or molasses is an eliminator and builder. The natural iron, copper, calcium, carbon, and hydrogen help build the blood to normal and give you plenty of energy. It truly is a perfect combination for cleansing, eliminating, and healing. Use for two days only.

Decongest Your Colon

A toxic colon can be caused by the following:

- Eating devitalized food
- Eating "The American way": Hamburgers, french fries, and a malt; macaroni and cheese; and, of course, the big culprit, white bread

The walls of the colon are constantly at work absorbing moisture out of the contents of the colon. The longer any material remains in the colon, the more dry and pressed together it becomes, and the glue coats the lining of the colon. This has been proven. When autopsies are performed, the lining of the colon is like hardened cement.

Our body is fed through the colon. When the colon is literally poisoned by a cesspool of decayed matter, the toxins released by the putrefactive process get into our bloodstream and travel to all parts of the body. Every cell in the body is affected, and many forms of sickness can result. The entire system is weakened. A toxic colon can be the causative factor for nearly any disease.

Illnesses due to toxic colons (asthma, hay fever, arteriosclerosis, cancer, arthritis, neuritis, hypertension, diabetes, etc.) are just manifestations of toxins that should escape through the lymphatic system. But, due to overload, the lymphatic system is unable to cleanse them, so mucoid substance settles in the lungs, muscles, tendons, and joints.

Because we are fed through the colon, this is where health and disease are determined. If a person has a toxic colon, all the good food and vitamins will have to pass through these toxins, lessening their nutritional value. The body becomes polluted: Its blood is only as clean as its intestinal tract, because it absorbs both nutritive and toxic materials from the colon. If a toxic colon is the underlying cause of many diseases, it makes sense that we should first choose to help ourselves by cleaning and decongesting our colon.

Here are several methods to cleanse your colon:

- Earl Irons method: Bentonite clay and cleanser for seven days
- An herbal combination of yellow dock, onion, sage, wahoo bark, and rhubarb root
- An herbal combination of white pine bark, mugwort, myrrh, chamomile, catnip, and mullein
- One tablespoon glycerin in one cup of coffee
- One quart lightly salted water upon rising

It's also important that your body process foods quickly to maintain health. Therefore, use the following suggestions to avoid constipation.

GENERAL RULES FOR RELIEVING CONSTIPATION

- Always drink plenty of pure water!

- Fresh fruits and vegetables are very important sources of roughage. Stewed vegetables and dried fruits are also helpful.

- Add unprocessed wheat bran and/or unprocessed wheat germ to your daily diet to normalize bowel function!

- Brewer's yeast is effective for many.

- Avoid excessive milk drinking.

- Daily morning or afternoon exercise (yoga, walking in fresh air, etc.).

- Go to the bathroom daily at the same time after a meal; relax, read there, stay awhile.

- Reflex massage stimulates the circulation of every gland in the body!

- Body massage and natural therapy improve circulation, digestion, respiration, organs of elimination, and the brain and nervous system (receive greater supply of blood).

Decongest Your Bowels with Flaxseed

Flaxseed must be gently simmered for about half an hour, then allowed to stand where it will remain hot for one to two hours. Put two tablespoons in two cups of boiling water and let it boil down to one cup. Add a little sugar to taste. The juice of half a lemon makes a tasty addition. Drink the whole cup at bedtime and swallow all the seeds. The mucilage is soothing to the bowels, and in combination with the seeds, often produces a good bowel movement. This combination is excellent to take about once a week or every four days—or more often if needed, since it is harmless.

Mucous Cleanser

This diet to clear mucous out of intestines was developed by a chiropractor in Los Angeles. It is amazing to see the amount of mucous leaving the body in people you never suspected had this trouble.

You need the following items:

- Unfiltered apple juice
- Psyllium seeds, Mucovada, or ground flaxseeds
- Papaya tablets
- Pancreatin
- Comfrey and pepsin
- Fenugreek seed

Combine the above ingredients as shown below:

- One glass distilled water with one teaspoon bulk (apple juice, seeds, and papaya tablets)
- One pancreatin
- One comfrey and pepsin
- One cup fenugreek seed tea

Follow this schedule every two hours from 7 A.M. until 9 P.M., and keep it up for three or four days. All mucous is cleansed, even from sinuses.

Decongest Your Joints: Arthritis

When arthritis sets in, one must adjust one's lifestyle, relying on a diet of equal parts raw and cooked food. Leave out sugar, cakes, cookies, potato chips, and heavy meals. Start exercising by swinging arms and legs. Bend your knees, and twist and stretch your body.

It is thought that most arthritis, osteoarthritis, and rheumatism have a hidden virus. In this country, the herbal antidote is a combination of yucca, black walnut leaves, yellow dock, wormwood, and fenugreek seed. These are used to repair the damage.

To help relieve arthritis, try the following remedies:

- Take one teaspoon cod-liver oil in orange juice at bedtime.
- Take one tablespoon almond oil in cherry juice upon rising. You can also use safflower oil or peanut oil.
- Take five to seven alfalfa juice tablets with each meal. Alfalfa releases the stiffness in joints and muscles.
- Take two glasses cherry juice or a saucer full of cherries a day. This counteracts uric acid.
- To rebuild the undernourished adrenal gland, which is so significant in arthritis, take licorice root, stress B with C, pantothenic acid, and take extra B_{12} and B_6 when the hands are affected. This will make the adrenal gland produce its own cortisone and other hormones. Omit coffee and sugar.
- Be sure that you take calcium with magnesium. Use two parts calcium and one part magnesium. This is a tranquilizer, a builder, a pain reliever, and an absolute must for all kinds of arthritic suffering. Take one-half of your calcium-magnesium intake with cod-liver oil.

Decongest Your Gallbladder

I have a book from the 17th century in which an old physician from Austria gives his secrets. One of them is the apple juice diet. This diet is used among health-minded people to detoxify the liver and gallbladder. One person told this story: "I had had a very bad summer. Too much work, too little sleep. I did not take food supplements and had to work under conditions where I had to eat fried foods and other no-no foods. In the fall it started. Tired, bloated, listless, I caught myself being sarcastic and nasty. One night I had terrible pain over my right shoulder and neck. I am sorry to say my liver quit her job, and the next morning I went on the apple juice diet. The bright green pebbles, the old bile, just poured out on the third day, and I was myself again."

This diet is recommended. Use it to give your gallbladder a rest, a holiday, and a chance.

First day:

8 A.M.	1 glass (8 oz.)	apple juice
10 A.M.	2 glasses (16 oz.)	apple juice
12 P.M.	2 glasses (16 oz.)	apple juice
2 P.M.	2 glasses (16 oz.)	apple juice
4 P.M.	2 glasses (16 oz.)	apple juice
6 P.M.	2 glasses (16 oz.)	apple juice

Juice should be natural—sugar and chemical free. No food is to be taken this day.

Second day:

Same procedure as the first day, again with no food. At bedtime take four ounces olive oil. You may wash the olive oil down with hot lemon juice or hot apple juice. Go to bed at once.

As a rule, this diet starts to work around 4 A.M. You will find little green pebbles in the fecal matter. They may be the size of a pinhead, or they may be as big as a bird egg. Many times it all looks like green mud. In any case, the old stagnant bile becomes dissolved and liquefied through the malic acid of the apple juice, and the oil helps remove the waste.

Dr. Adolphus Hohensee has been using this diet on thousands of his students all over America. In Europe it is practiced in health spas and hospitals with equal results. It reestablishes the normal function of the liver. This diet frees the liver-gallbladder tract from old bile and debris—which we call stones!

Decongest Your Eyes: Glaucoma

What follows is a three-month program that entails a very low carbohydrate diet and no sugar or coffee (or very, very weak coffee).

First month:
100,000 IU vitamin A once daily (half from beta carotene and half from fish oil)
20 mg. B-complex before each meal
25 mg. B_2 before each meal
Coffee enema once daily
Chop a large onion once daily for a good cry

Second month:
75,000 IU vitamin A (half from beta carotene and half from fish oil)
No coffee enema
The rest is the same as the first month

Third month:
50,000 IU vitamin A (half from beta carotene and half from fish oil).
The rest is the same as the second month

To combat congestion of the eyes, combine the juices of half a potato, half a cucumber, half an onion, and one-quarter of a pepper. Drink six ounces of this a half hour before supper, and watch your eyes get cleaner after thirty days.

Decongest Your Kidneys

A great deal of attention should be paid to the kidneys. A sick kidney does not hurt until the sickness expands to the outer encasing. Then it hurts badly, especially when stones pass through the kidney ducts.

A sick kidney presses upwards. It causes a stiff neck, disk trouble, stiff and painful arms, back problems, and fuzzy eyesight. In advanced cases, kidney problems manifest in sore knees and, finally, swollen ankles. Two-thirds of all people committed to mental institutions have kidney disorders. If patients become wild or disoriented, the kidneys should be checked.

The right kidney is the organ that filters inorganic substances, such as toxic lead, mercury, copper, DDT, and arsenic-bound chemicals. When overloaded, this organ does not hurt, but becomes cold to the touch. The left kidney is sensitive to infections.

To cleanse the kidneys, consume an eight-ounce glass of raw beet juice, taking it one teaspoon at a time throughout the day. Don't eat anything that day. Water is allowed. The urine turns red as the system absorbs the beet juice drop by drop. A day of this every six months truly uses food as a medicine.

Decongest Your Kidneys from Stones

Dr. Christian Chaussy, a compassionate German research urologist, presented a paper to the American Urological Association in Boston, reporting on 72 kidney stone cases in which he and his group had successfully pulverized the stones extracorporeally, without resorting to surgery. Unfortunately, we have been unable to find any place in the United States where stones from high in the ureter can be removed safely without surgery.

Small wonder that Dr. Chaussy's research facility, which is subsidized by grants from the German government, cannot begin to accept all of the patients from around the world who write, asking to be accepted into his program. Dr. Chaussy does on occasion, however, take patients from other countries. His grant covers work only on stones in the kidney, not in the ureter.

It is important to drink plenty of fluids—especially in warm weather—if you have ever had or think you might have a tendency to form kidney stones. Adults should drink enough to produce two to two and a half liters of urine every day. (Measure your output—about five pints, or ten cups—until you are sure your intake is sufficient to assure this large volume of urine.)

The *American Journal of Medicine*, Volume 71, October 1981, said, "The efficacy of thiazide and allopurinol in the prevention of calcium stones has long been established in large series of patients with renal calculi (1-3). However, at the customary dosage of hydrochlorothiazide, 50 mg. twice a day, the incidence of side effects (such as hypokalemia, extracellular volume depletion, hyperuricemia, weakness, fatigue and mental irritability) may necessitate discontinuation of treatment in a significant proportion (10 to 35 percent) of patients (1, 4)."

For kidney stones, take seven ounces dark grape juice and add one-half teaspoon cream of tartar. Take two ounces three times daily before meals, and drink one quart of the following tea daily: Equal parts knotgrass and chamomile. Keep it up for five weeks. Drink a little all day long, and do not ice it!

Stone and Gout Remedy

To relieve symptoms, combine 1 tsp. hydrangea root and 1 qt. apple cider. Let these stand for 12 hours, bring to a boil, simmer, and drink one-half cup three times daily.

Also, take 15 to 20 sour cherries every morning for three weeks.

Decongest Your Lymphatic System

Try the following recipes to relieve symptoms.

Recipe No. 1:
1 pt. white grapefruit juice
1 pt. freshly squeezed orange juice
1 pt. grape juice
1 pt. water with the juice of 3 limes
1 pt. water with the juice of 2 lemons
1 pt. frozen pineapple juice, diluted
1 pt. papaya juice, diluted
12 whole eggs
6 egg yolks

Frozen raspberries or strawberries add a delicious flavor. Beat eggs and mix into fruit juice mixture. This is one day's supply. If you are hungry, add one kind of fresh fruit. For lunch, eat a green salad and/or sprouts with raw almond dressing. For supper, have a green salad and/or sprouts with raw almond dressing and one steamed vegetable.

Recipe No. 2:
Drink four to five cups of cucumber juice daily for one week. It purifies the lymphatic system and the blood, and it clears the complexion.

Recipe No. 3:
Boil three tablespoons barley in one quart water for 30 minutes. Add a little clove and cinnamon. Drink this in one day. It will clear the congestion in the lymphatic system.

Recipe No. 4:
1 pt. apple juice or apple wine
1 pt. water
1 pt. milk

Heat slowly and do not bring to a boil. When it curdles, strain it through a fine cloth, throw curds away and sweeten with honey if needed. Take two tablespoons five times daily if the person is very weak. Appetite will soon return. As the patient gets stronger, give up to two cups daily. It is powerful.

Decongest Your Liver

The liver is the most affected organ when it comes to metal and chemical poisoning. You have to clean our your liver—old debris can include metals such as lead, mercury, or arsenic; chemicals such as DDT; and so on.

A liver flush is indicated every time that you have the following symptoms:

- You start to ache without reason.
- You touch your right collarbone on the knob and it is painful to touch.
- You become disenchanted with life.
- You find fault with your neighbor.
- You are comfortable with dark glasses.

Then it is time to clean your liver. Buy large cans of stewed tomatoes. It's better to make your own, but do not add any fat. Eat as much as you can and also drink tomato juice.

It is amazing how hungry you become, so at bedtime on the second day you will look forward to the following cocktail:

3 oz. olive oil
2 oz. castor oil
3 oz. whip cream

Stir and drink this before bed when you are relaxed and ready for sleep. You may chew a little piece of lemon afterwards just for taste. At 3 A.M. or 4 A.M. you will experience nature's call, resulting in elimination of toxins from the body. The next morning, have what you want for breakfast.

Accumulation of toxins in the body may occur due to failure of the detoxification systems—liver, kidney, thyroid, adrenals, and colon. Accumulation may also be due to faulty metabolism or toxic matter at large.

Decongest Your Liver and Pancreas

Soak one pound dried apricots in pineapple juice overnight. Next morning, blend it and add fresh pineapple pieces and juice so that it becomes thick enough to spoon it. Divide it into four portions and eat it morning, noon, night, and bedtime, preferably not eating anything else that day. *Do not use if you are a diabetic.*

Decongest Your Spleen

The spleen is the reservoir in which the body's electricity is stored. If the spleen is not in order, the brain takes over this job. However, it has one drawback. People become egocentric. They accomplish nothing worthwhile.

Okra and red beets are revitalizing foods for the spleen.

Recipe:

Two qts. concord grape juice
Juice of six oranges
Juice of three lemons

Cut the white of the lemon into small pieces. Boil this in a little water for ten minutes. Add water to the drink. Then take distilled water and fill the liquid mixture to one gallon. This is one day's supply of your food-drink intake. Just two days of this will cleanse your organs.

Decongest Your Skin

To cleanse tissues: Make yourself six ounces of fresh orange juice ten times daily. Add two ounces of distilled water and drink slowly. Drink a hot tea made from wood sanicle and peppermint three times daily, that is, morning, noon, and night. No food.

After two to three days, your skin will be different. The calcium deposits in your body will be lessened due to the lime in the oranges. You may continue the orange juice another three days, but eat apples, pears, berries, and cottage cheese, also.

Decongest Your Stomach

"A sick stomach makes crippled, stiff hands." For sick stomachs—for ulcers, pain, discomfort, and suffering from stomach distress—the following foods are particularly healing:

- Carrots
- Coconut milk
- Eggplant
- Flaxseed tea
- Slippery elm tea with cream
- Goat's milk
- Okra
- Egg whites
- Parsnip
- Sweet potatoes
- Cottage cheese
- Aloe vera juice (best of all)

No grapefruit for stomach-troubled people.

If you are anxious to be healed from stomach ulcers, try the carrot diet. Boil a good quantity of carrots in pure water, such as artesian. Avoid aluminum of any kind, whether found in pots, pans, or foil. After the carrots are done, try them in various ways. Take a napkin and eat them rabbit style. Mash them or puree them. Boil them after they are cooked or make a soup of them. Slice them lengthwise or in squares. No butter or salt may be added. This is all you eat for seven days. Twice daily you may have six ounces of raw carrot juice, either with two tablespoons of cream, or with six ounces of goat's milk.

Decongest Your Stomach from Mucous

Mucous cleansers of the stomach are taken in the following manner: One glass fresh orange juice, same amount of distilled water. Do not mix. First drink the orange juice, then follow with the water. Do this as often as you want, ten times daily or so. No other food should be taken. Do it two days in a row two to three times a year.

High-Fiber Diet

The main function of fiber in a diet is to normalize the transit of food through the digestive system, allowing efficient elimination of waste. To quote one author, "We've been around for 3.5 million years thriving on a high-fiber diet for all but the last 50 years. And this is beginning to show with dramatic increases in a wide variety of diseases, from heart disease to colon cancer." The list includes the diverticular diseases: Hemorrhoids, appendicitis, ulcerative colitis, and constipation. Physicians find that when more fiber-rich food is eaten, these diseases tend to disappear.

Dr. Andrew Stanway, former chief physician at King's College Hospital in London and a nutrition expert, explains, "The swift movement of bran (and other fibers) through the body means that cancer-causing agents have less time to start the processes leading to colon cancer. This fast movement also prevents conditions such as gallstones, stomach ailments, and circulatory problems."

Dr. Siegel, author of *Dr. Siegel's Natural Fiber Permanent Weight-Loss Diet* and whose clinics have successfully used a high-fiber diet with patients, says that "A high-bran diet with few refined carbohydrates will safely take pounds off and keep them off."

Dr. Emanuel Cheraskin of the University of Alabama Dental School, author of 13 books on the relationship between diet and disease, says a high-fiber diet will help prevent heart disease, colon cancer, gallstones, stomach ailments, hemorrhoids, and blood clots.

When we think of fiber food, we think of bran. Yes, it is the richest food in fiber; however, it has a drawback. The sharp edges of the bran may injure the already sick colon. To avoid injury, add wheat germ to your bran. Wheat germ is also high in fiber and has some health-giving, vitamin-E-rich oils in it that lubricate the bran. Wheat germ reduces the danger of bran bulking in the intestines.

Raw and cooked vegetables, whole grain breads, fruit, berries, beans, and corn all have fibers and will keep a healthy colon at its best. Once a colon is sick, weakened, or diseased, special care and diets must be utilized.

Recent findings tell us that fiber "is the important thing." Formerly, we were told not to use fiber because it might cause a variety of colon troubles. Where is the truth?

The truth is in the wholeness of food. The carrot and the whole potato have fiber, and the grains have bran. Hidden in this natural fiber are minerals that we will not get if we eat only a part of the wholeness. Consider the following daily intake:

- Protein drink for breakfast
- Doughnut and coffee for a snack
- Soft bread and soft cheese for lunch
- A small salad for supper with mashed potatoes and meat
- Cakes and cookies for dessert

There is just not enough fiber!

Bran, a natural food fiber, is tasteless and easy to take. Mix three tablespoons bran and three tablespoons raw or toasted wheat germ. Add it to any kind of food you want—from soup to cereals to ground beef.

Nerves

The following routine, performed only three days in a row, will make you a stronger personality. After that, one day a week or one day every two weeks will keep your nerves sweet.

In one pint of cottage cheese, mix three tablespoons almond oil or safflower oil and two egg yolks. Mix well, and either make the mixture sweet with honey or spicy with onions, salt, and herbs. Also boil four tablespoons of barley in two quarts of water for 35 minutes. Strain, and add honey or lime or lemon juice to the barley water so it tastes good.

Before breakfast:	One cup of warm barley water
Breakfast:	Prepared cottage cheese and carrots, raw or cooked
Mid-morning:	Barley water
Noon:	Steamed zucchini, cooked green beans, and cottage cheese (spicy)
Mid-afternoon:	Barley water
Evening:	Prepared cottage cheese, zucchini (stewed or baked in the oven), dish of barley, carrot salad, and barley water
Bedtime:	Barley water and calcium tablets

Pregnancy

Dr. V. Noodan estimated that the needed caloric intake of a fetus during pregnancy between the second and fifth months is 150 calories, and later on, 300 to 400 calories over the needs of the mother. That is not very much. However, the quality of the food is important.

When we speak of quality, we think of proteins, but in pregnancy, this is not the way to go. The unborn needs minerals, such as calcium, iron, magnesium, zinc, and the whole range of trace minerals—organic and inorganic. For instance, it was calculated that the fetus needs 34 grams of pure calcium to develop properly. If there is not enough calcium, the new developing body will rob calcium from the mother's body. If during pregnancy a mother refrains from salt, she can drink all the fluids she wants without causing edema.

The following recipe has helped many from pregnancy intoxications: Take one level teaspoon Epsom salts in six ounces water every hour, four times. That will relieve the danger at once.

Whenever albumin shows in the urine of the mother, milk should no longer be given. Diluted fruit juices, water, and vegetable juices are to be taken.

The normal development of the child is dependent on the presence of enough vitamins, such as A, B-complex, C-complex, D, and E. One hundred IU of vitamin E is a must. Vitamin A is absorbed best through carrots.

Therefore, during pregnancy, every woman should have vitamin and mineral supplements, good natural foods, vegetables and fruits, and whole grains. A natural-food diet is the best assurance against miscarriages and makes for a happy pregnancy.

Phlebitis

Use the following methods to relieve phlebitis symptoms:

- Eat sparingly. Drink plenty of diluted fruit or vegetable juices—six ounces juice to two ounces water. No meat, cheese, or egg allowed.

- Make a tea of two parts white oak bark, one and a half parts St. John's wort, and two parts yarrow. Drink one quart cool tea daily and also apply cool tea to the leg.

- Drink six ounces aloe vera juice over the course of a day and eat two tablespoons blackstrap molasses daily.
- Two tablespoons maple syrup, one glass of water, and a dash of red root or paprika. Drink half a glass every hour for one day or more.

~⚜ CHAPTER FOUR ⚜~

Metals and Other Poisons As a Cause of Ill Health

No machine can be overhauled while the components are in motion. Before an engine can be repaired or totally overhauled, all movement of its parts must cease. Unlike the machine, our bodies are endowed with the ability to store sufficient energy to function for considerable time without fuel intake, and it is during these periods that nature can heal your body best.

In the past, many concerned professionals became dissatisfied with methods used in orthodox medicine, with the many, many side effects of drug therapy (which truly is a shock therapy—"shocking the system into balance"). These men and women instructed us to follow the path of nontoxic methods.

However, in their lifetime they did not face catastrophic environmental pollution such as atomic fallout, lead poisoning (gasoline), arsenic poisoning (spray), or sodium fluoride poisoning (drinking water). In those times, our population did not have the breakdown of the immune system due to poisons, EHF waves, ELF waves, microwaves, computers, and televisions. These were unknown. We are confronted with a totally different situation today, and we have to do our utmost to keep our families, our communities, and our world healthy.

If you realize that no section of society is free from the drug menace (even our athletes come under its influence), you will agree that we have to stand up and protect ourselves and our offspring. We live in a poisoned, chemically treacherous world. We cannot change this, but we can help ourselves so that environmental poisons such as lead, arsenic, chemicals, and pollution do not harm us. We have to answer the following questions:

- Where are the poisons?
- What harm do they do?
- How do we recognize them?
- How do we eliminate them?

Aluminum Poisoning

Concerned health practitioners in the United States and Canada are urging their patrons to avoid products containing aluminum. Why? Aluminum has a predisposition to affect neuronal tissue. Many tests done on animals showed that behavior and memory suffered as aluminum levels were increased in lymph and brain.

Many researchers feel that aluminum is the major culprit in Alzheimer's disease, a disease of dementia, forgetfulness, and senility. Autopsies showed that individuals afflicted with Alzheimer's disease had accumulated six times as much aluminum in the brain as healthy people.

I urge you not to take a chance. Throw away your aluminum pots, and beverages in aluminum containers. Dr. Berlyne, Ben Ari, and others stated, "The practice of cooking in aluminum utensils and wrapping foods in aluminum foil may result in gross changes in the aluminum content of food before ingestion." Aluminum is also found in the following products:

- Antacids
- Toothpaste
- Baking powder
- Antiperspirants

Also, numerous cities add aluminum salt to drinking water to reduce its cloudiness. This also makes the water cosmetically pleasing.

The following symptoms may indicate aluminum poisoning:

- Dryness of mouth
- Stomach ulcers
- Forgetfulness
- Hard stool and/or small hardened pieces or "feces stones"
- Stomach pain
- Pain in spleen area
- Children who cry a lot
- Kidney problems, especially the right kidney

What to Do

Antidote No. 1: Use homeopathic *Alumina* 6x to 12x.

Antidote No. 2: Use this herbal combination: Pumpkin seed, okra, rhubarb root, capsicum, peppermint, and dulse.

Antidote No. 3: Find coenzyme minerals in an aqueous extraction of naturally chelated colloidal minerals. These minerals are derived from an ancient seabed mineral deposit. The action of colloidal aluminum with other enzymes removes aluminum deposits on the order of God's law that "like attracts like."

Many illnesses, including good or bad tumors, are in the end aluminum accumulations. By removing and transmuting aluminum, the body can rid itself of all kinds of troubles.

Arsenic Poisoning

Many household and garden pesticides contain arsenoxide. Acute arsenic poisoning has to be treated at once in the emergency room, and this is not the place to discuss it. However, chronic arsenic poisoning is rarely discovered and hardly ever discussed.

Here are the chronic arsenic poisoning symptoms:

- Sweetish metallic taste
- Garlicky odor to breath and stool
- Constriction of throat
- Difficulties in swallowing
- Burning pains in esophagus, stomach, and sometimes bowels
- Muscle spasms
- Pain in muscles of back
- Spine is pulled out of line so that people have to go for adjustments over and over again (adjustments do not hold). (Elkium and Faky said that the element arsenic is an active enzyme inhibitor.)

- Mild gastrointestinal disturbances
- Anorexia
- Low-grade fever (changes in white blood count)
- Weakness
- Catarrhal symptoms (nose, throat, eyes)
- Brittle nails
- Loss of hair
- Localized edema in the eyelids signifies problems in the liver, possibly due to arsenic
- Nervousness

Because arsenic has a constricting effect on the muscle structure and lodges in muscles, the most outstanding symptom is a constant backache.

Arsenic also settles in the brain, dislodging the phosphorus that is needed for proper brain functioning.

What to Do

If you can find Mexican raw sugar, take one teaspoon three times daily. Homeopathic *Arsenicum metallicum* 6x also does the job. The herbal combination of pumpkin seed, okra, rhubarb root, capsicum, peppermint, and dulse transmutes almost all metals.

Very helpful is the herb from southern and eastern Africa called *Harpagophytum procumbens* (devil's claw). This tea washes out metallic poisons as well as chemical poisons. It carries the rare combination of three active ingredients: Flukoside, fruran, and pyror.

There is also an old-time natural remedy used over centuries that can be found in the book *Biochemical Toxicology* by Ernest Hodgson and Frank Guthrie.

Cadmium Poisoning[1]

Although cadmium is found in foods, the levels are too low to be of any toxicological significance. Cadmium has many industrial uses—for example,

---
[1] Nordberg, G.F. (Ed.) "Effects and Dose-response Relationships of Toxic Metals." Amsterdam: Elsevier, 1976; Symposium on biological and pharmacological effects of metal contaminants. Fed. Proc. 27 (1977), 15.

electroplating, low-melting alloys, low friction, fatigue-resistant bearing alloys, solders, batteries, pigments, and a barrier in atomic fission control. Therefore, it is to be expected that low to moderate cadmium content of the environment is widespread. Since chronic exposure to even low levels of trace elements can lead to health problems, cadmium is of particular importance to those concerned with environmental quality.

Industrial exposure is the most prevalent cause of chronic and acute cadmium toxicity. Chronic toxicity is manifested in humans by anosmia (loss of the sense of smell) as a result of olfactory nerve damage, kidney dysfunction, and emphysema. Cadmium has also been implicated as a possible cause of lung cancer. The cadmium content of tobacco leaves is significant, but there is no experimental evidence linking cadmium in tobacco to emphysema and lung cancer. It has been suggested that cadmium may play a role in the production of arteriosclerosis, hypertension, and cardiovascular disease, but the data are limited and contradictory. It is worth noting that the body's burden of cadmium in smokers is one and a half to two times that of nonsmokers.

Acute cadmium toxicity in humans often leads to pneumonitis, ranging from severe to fatal. Vomiting, diarrhea, and prostration are also symptoms of acute cadmium poisoning.

Cadmium affects the activities of several enzymes. Enhanced activity of Δ-amino levulinic acid dehydratase, pyruvate dehydrogenase, and pyruvate decarboxylase have been noted, while depressed activity of Δ-amino levulinic acid synthetase, alcohol dehydrogenase, aryl sulfatase, and lipoamide dehydrogenase result from cadmium intoxication.

Cadmium has been shown to interact with phospholipids, such as phosphatidylserine and phosphatidylethanolamine. These interactions may be responsible for the toxic effects of cadmium on membranes.

Cadmium settles predominantly in the heart and right kidney.

Cadmium poisoning may be alleviated through:

- More zinc intake
- More paprika
- Homeopathic *Cadmium metallicum* in low potency (6x to 30x)

Lead Poisoning

Lead is still one of the more commonly used toxic heavy metals, but its modern use is not nearly so diverse as it was during the 17th through the 19th centuries. The gastrointestinal absorption of lead varies with age; adults absorb 5 to 10 percent of an oral dose, whereas children may absorb up to 50 percent of an oral dose. Lead is stored in the liver and bone—particularly bone—where it accumulates over a period of many years, if not throughout the lifetime. Lead is particularly detrimental to children, who store it in the coverings of the bones and joints. It has an affinity for the lipoids and stores in the nervous system and in the brain.

Exposure to lead takes on many forms in addition to that of industrial hazards. Although lead intake from paints, water pipes, tin cans, and insecticides has decreased, exposure to other forms of lead, such as in motor vehicle exhausts and tobacco smoke, has either stabilized or increased. Intake of lead paint by children is still a problem in poor urban neighborhoods where painted surfaces may still contain lead. Lead poisoning has been reported in the southern United States as a result of the consumption of nontaxed, distilled alcoholic beverages—commonly known as moonshine.

On windless days, you can see the car exhaust lingering over our highways. In a long gray-blue strip it lies there like a monster. In fact, it is a monster that consumes our health. When lead is taken in through the lungs, it is more likely to be in suspension in the fluids of the body, such as the lymphatic fluid, the blood, and the gland fluids. When eaten with food as the Romans did, it is more likely to be deposited in the joints, liver, pancreas, and heart.

It is said that the fall of Rome was nothing more than accumulated lead poisoning in all of its citizens. They used to carry their water in lead pipes and lead containers, and the accumulated lead destroyed the nation. Our water pipes are safe, but how about the air we breathe? Are the cities and the crowded highways safe?

Symptoms of lead poisoning include abdominal pain, anemia, and lesions of the central and peripheral nervous systems. The lesions of the central nervous system cause behavioral problems. The anemia is characterized by a larger than normal number of erythrocytes and is of the hypochromic, microcytic type.

The principal biochemical effect of lead intoxication in humans and animals is defective hemoglobin synthesis. Lead inhibits iron incorporation into protoporphyrin, which results in lower heme concentrations and higher protoporphyrin concentrations in erythrocytes. Excretion of coproporphyrin is increased, and the iron content of the blood plasma and bone marrow is elevated. Lead also interferes with an earlier step in heme synthesis by inhibiting Δ-amino levulinic acid dehydratase, which converts Δ-amino levulinic acid to prophobilinogen. The resulting increase of Δ-amino levulinic acid in blood and urine is a sensitive indicator of lead poisoning (also known as *plumbism*). In advanced lead poisoning, synthesis of the globin moiety of hemoglobin is also inhibited.

Lead is a protoplasmic poison. That means it interferes with the proper life-energy-enzyme exchange in the living body. It is amazing how beautifully our system is able to take this load of lead poisoning. Everyone has it. Only a few people in very isolated places in the mountains or prairies are free from lead intoxication.

We need to consider the amount of lead in our system and our tolerance factor for lead, arsenic, cadmium, mercury, copper, and other heavy metals. This tolerance factor differs in everyone. Some people sponge in more arsenic than others, some more lead, some more aluminum-lead, and some more mercury. I've found redheaded people are prone to take in more copper than others. Asian people take in more mercury. Fair-complected people take in more lead and aluminum. The individual tolerance also differs widely. In every case of leukemia, the tolerance level of arsenic should be checked. In every case of exhaustion, the lead level should be checked.

The Biologisch-Physicalische Research Institute in Obergensingen, Germany, reports that the lead contamination of the atmosphere is increasingly alarming. Every third patient shows lead poisoning. Most probably the car exhaust is at fault. Every gallon of gasoline contains 60 mg. of lead. Approximately 8,000 tons of this lead are puffed into the atmosphere every year. In the streets, children and small animals are particularly exposed to the dangers of poisons through heavy metal accumulations in the atmosphere, because these metals have a tendency to settle down.

The scientists of Obergensingen developed an instrument that enables them to test 1,000 blood samples a day. They are trying to find an antidote to the accumulations of lead residue in humans and animals. Their findings are widely publicized in an effort to change the condition of air pollution at least in their country.

The lead problems in our country and all civilized countries started in 1922 when Mighty and Boyd added lead ethyl to gasoline. The balance quota of lead in America is 0.002 mg./m³, which can be 60 times as high in rush-hour traffic. Out of 5 to 10 percent of dust that the lung takes in, 50 percent of it is lead dust.

Lead poisoning can interfere with enzyme processes by displacing the essential mineral nucleus or by precipitating (gluing) the enzymes together. Because of the changes in the biochemistry of the body due to heavy metal toxins, it is extremely important to take an extra supply of essential minerals.

The most serious manifestation is lead encephalopathy, which requires prompt and skillful treatment. Increased intracranial pressure may occur suddenly and must be treated vigorously. Encephalopathy is very serious. It causes a mortality rate of 25 percent or more, and it often leaves mental retardation and various permanent neurological lesions in those who sur-vive. In adults, permanent blindness, extraocular muscle paralysis, or other lesions may result. The acute form caused by tetraethyl lead is either fatal or followed by complete recovery. There is great urgency in beginning treat-ment of this form. One cannot wait to get the results of lead analysis before starting treatment.

Scientific Studies of Lead and Mercury Levels in Emotionally Disturbed Children

Children exposed to toxic amounts of lead and other metal pollutants are subject to severe behavioral disorders resulting from damage to the central nervous system (Byers and Lord, 1943; Pfeiffer, 1977). It remains to be determined whether subtoxic metal levels are an etiologic agent in behavioral disorders. Subtoxic lead levels previously thought harmless are now being associated with hyperactivity, impulsiveness, short attention span, and immaturity.

In Wyoming, an outstanding examination was made of schoolchildren with learning and behavioral problems. After obtaining parental permission, researchers asked children to submit a small sample of hair (about 400 mg.) for trace minerals analysis. The senior researcher collected hair samples from the nape of each child's neck, as close to the scalp as possible, using stainless steel scissors. The hair samples were submitted to a state-licensed clinical laboratory where they were analyzed with three instruments—the atomic absorption spectrophotometer, the graphite furnace, and the induction-coupled plasma torch—to determine five toxic metal levels. The five toxic metal levels tested for were lead, mercury, arsenic, cadmium, and aluminum. Precise laboratory techniques were used to assure reliability requirements. The two groups of children showed the following results.

Metal Group	Emotionally disturbed children	Control
Lead	10.78 parts per million (ppm)	2.76 ppm
Mercury	1.30 ppm	.47 ppm
Arsenic	2.74 ppm	1.35 ppm
Cadmium	.75 ppm	.37 ppm
Aluminum	12.62 ppm	.00 ppm

The data of this study do not establish a causative relationship, but they do show an association between lead and mercury concentrations and behavioral deficiency in children.

The neurochemical studies of Dr. Silbergeld and Houshka (1980) showed that lead and mercury are potent neurotoxins. Their effects are demonstrated in the neuronal system by using tests with acetylcholine, catecholamines, and gamma-aminobutyric acid (GABA) as transmitters.

Looking back to the toxic metal chart, you will notice that the aluminum level of disturbed children is very high, while it's nonexistent in the control group. In my personal opinion, this has to be noted, and further study needs to be done to verify findings.

These studies are very important, and scientists caution us not to assume that there is a "safe" level of lead and mercury exposure; there is concern that neurons may be irreversibly damaged by an exposure to lead and also mercury.

When lead is being stored in the nervous system, the following symptoms are observed:

- Mad, weakened constitution
- Lack of willpower
- Lack of abstract thinking ability

- Tooth decay
- Allergic reactions to food and environment

Lead is stored in the kidneys, liver, bone marrow, and spleen. This causes an increase in diabetes, multiple sclerosis, tooth decay, and a lack of mental capacity.

What to Do

You are the only one who can do something about it. Here are some recipes to help detoxify the body.

First method:
2 qts. cranberry juice
3 tsp. whole cloves
2 tsp. ground cinnamon
1 tsp. cream of tartar

Boil the cloves in one quart cranberry juice for 20 minutes. Strain and add two teaspoons ground cinnamon. Stir and add it to the rest of the cranberry juice. Now add one teaspoon cream of tartar. Stir. Drink eight ounces three times daily for 12 to 15 days. For children, six ounces two times daily for 12 to 15 days. Then, do it once a week.

Second method:
This is a wonderful herbal formula for taking out lead residue: Combine six ounces basil, one ounce rosemary, one ounce hyssop, and one ounce boneset.

Third method:
Try the following herbal combination: Pumpkin seed, okra, rhubarb root, capsicum, peppermint, and dulse.

Fourth method:
A combination of cloves and vitamin C will combat the problem of lead in the body. Researchers and doctors have made numerous statements about

the terrible effects of lead in the tissues, indicating that it is everywhere, and almost everyone has some lead deposits. It has been found that cloves and vitamin C do an excellent job of neutralizing this widespread situation. Also, some colds and flu respond to this combination.

Mercury Poisoning

Edmund B. Fink indicates that many features of poisoning by heavy metals are similar, but the important metals from the standpoint of toxicology are arsenic, lead, mercury, and others. You may review his findings in his book, *Diseases Due to Chemical Factors*, where he says that Mercury occurs as a bright, shining, silver white metal, liquid at ordinary temperatures, and easily divisible into globules. Mercury has a specific gravity of about 13.5. Mercury is insoluble in the ordinary solvents, in hydrochloric acid, and at ordinary temperatures in sulfuric acid, but it is soluble in the latter upon boiling. It is readily and completely soluble in nitric acid.

Since mercury ion precipitates protein, mercuric salts are protoplasmic poisons, and metallic mercury and its various compounds are at least potentially so. The toxicity and often the action of mercury compounds are proportional to the content of mercuric ion. Mercury and its salts and other compounds have been variously used as antiseptics, parasiticides, fungicides, antiluetic agents, diuretics, and catharsis.

Absorption and Elimination

Metallic mercury in bulk is not absorbed, but when it is dispersed in very small globules having a large total surface area or when it is present in the form of a salt or of certain other compounds, it is absorbed by the mucosa of the alimentary tract. It is also absorbed through the skin and by inhalation as vapor. Mercury is excreted chiefly through the kidneys and the colon, although it has been detected in practically every secretion of the body, including sweat, bile, and milk. Elimination is comparatively slow. While most of a dose of mercury is excreted during the first week, the excretion nevertheless continues for months. Intake of as little as 0.4 mg. of mercury daily may result in poisoning.

The equivalent of 500 mg. of mercury was found in the liver and kidneys of a man who had not received treatment for several months before his death. It was also found in the spleen, intestinal walls, heart, skeletal muscles, lungs, and bones. When present in blood in higher concentrations, it acts as a local irritant and leads to increased glandular secretion. The salivary glands are the most sensitive, so that ptyalism is an early symptom of chronic mercury poisoning; however, the kidneys and bowels are affected also.

Mercury was the first antisyphilitic drug that had real therapeutic action, but it is no longer used for that purpose. At one time mercurials were highly regarded for their antiphlogistic (anti-inflammatory) action in the treatment of inflammations of membranes as in pleurisy, iritis, and peritonitis, especially when the exudate was of a fibrinous nature.

Edmund Fink writes, "Mercury ions even in fairly diluted solutions denature protein and cause protein precipitation. Mercury poisoning can make damage to the basal ganglia of the brain, which can induce Parkinson-like symptoms."

The term *erethism* is applied to the psychic disturbance characterized by irritability, shyness, and deterioration of family and social activities, suggesting mercury or other metal poisoning.

Since makers of felt hats formerly used mercury salts in the manufacturing process and often became "mad," these symptoms gave rise to the phrase, "mad as a hatter."

The following symptoms indicate chronic mercury poisoning:

- Salivation is excessive and there is a metallic taste in the mouth.
- A blue line develops along the gingival margin.
- Gums become hypertrophied, bleed easily, and are sore.
- Teeth become loose.
- Tremors of the eyelids, lips, tongue, fingers, and extremities are characteristic of chronic poisoning.
- Coarse, jerky movements and gross incoordination interfere with fine movements such as writing and eating.
- Atrophy of the cerebellar cortex and, to a lesser extent, of the cerebral cortex occurs.
- Microscopic changes occur in the granular layer of the cerebellum, ganglion cells, and posterior columns.

Mercurial Intoxication

Ethyl and methyl compounds of mercury are used for fungal diseases of cereals and grain. These compounds have an affinity for the central nervous system and produce the following:

- Generalized ataxia
- Eczema, allergy
- Insomnia
- Tremors
- Anxiety, mental depression
- Loss of hearing

- Deafness
- Progressive visual deterioration
- Suicidal tendency
- Loss of coordination
- Loss of memory
- Coma and death

Changes in the central nervous system similar to the lesions of chronic mercury poisoning are found.

Hypersensitivity reactions to mercurial diuretic agents include asthma, urticaria, exfoliative dermatitis, and sudden death.

Kidney trouble such as proteinuria and nephrotic syndrome has been caused by contact with ammoniated mercury and other compounds.

What to Do

In the case of environmental metallic poisoning from metals such as lead, arsenic, aluminum, mercury, and so on, try the following diet, which relieves the body of environmental poisons. Use this diet when metals are lodged in your glands and nerves.

Three-Day Diet:
3 lbs. green beans
2 lbs. celery
4 lbs. zucchini
3 bunches parsley

Boil the green beans in plenty of water until done. Add finely chopped celery and coarsely cut zucchini. Boil another five minutes or until the zucchini is done. Remove from heat and add three bunches of finely chopped parsley. Season with spice or another herb flavor. This is all you eat—and all you will want—for the next three days. Eat this until it is all gone. Make more if needed. When reheating, take only a portion from the refrigerator and eat all you want. Eat the mixture as often as you want. Drink parsley tea or willow leaf tea as a beverage.

Eat more iron and more calcium foods.

Antidotes to Metallic Poisons

Vitamin C is needed to counteract environmental poisons. Dr. Linus Pauling stated that vitamin C stimulates interferon production. Interferon is needed to strengthen the immune system.

Pectin from citrus binds metals to some extent. Eat the whole fruit.

Pollen, a quarter teaspoon twice daily, has proven to bind environmental poisons.

Lead—Green beans and zucchini should be eaten exclusively for three days. This will get rid of metallic poisons.

Aluminum and arsenic—Squash removes arsenic poisons. Strawberries are extra good for smokers. They also remove other metallic poisons.

Arsenic—Mexican raw sugar removes arsenic poisons. Take one teaspoon several times daily until symptoms subside.

Plutonium, strontium 90, cadmium, calcium, and mercury poisons—Algae are a terrific help in counteracting environmental poisons. Red algae bind plutonium poison. Brown algae bind strontium 90 and cadmium poisons. Green algae bind calcium and mercury poisons.

Lead—Chamomile is very helpful to drink for lead poisoning and is soothing to the nerves. It has a lot of calcium in it, so it is very good for young children, especially in getting them to replace the lead with calcium in the body.

Strontium 90 + Cesium

These came into our lives through nuclear testing. Strontium 90 may be nullified by the intake of biological calcium as calcium orotate, calcium phosphate (cell salt #2), and calcium sulfate (cell salt #3). See Cell Salts, in chapter 1.

Sulfur Baths

One of the most universal remedies to remove lead, arsenic, platinum, gold, and mercury from your body is sulfur baths. The sulfur baths in Europe are overcrowded. Many Americans find help there. Every summer a stream of Americans fly to European spas to take care of their health problems. Yet, we have these wonderful healing waters right here in this country. They are undiscovered and unattended. The precious water runs into the beautiful wilderness. A national campaign should be started to build beautiful spas around these precious sulfur waters. It should be made available to rich and poor alike.

Thanks to the advances of industry, sulfur baths are available in dry form, and the granules, tablets, or powders can be added to our bathwater once a month.

Cranberry juice is also very good for removing toxins from the body. A suggested way is four ounces cranberry juice and four ounces distilled water. Take this mixture four times daily for three days, then wait about five days and repeat. About 120 units of toxins can be eliminated daily with this program.

Toxic Metals

The following chart summarizes the important facts about five toxic metals—aluminum, arsenic, cadmium, lead, and mercury—showing you how they affect you, where they come from, and how you can cleanse yourself.

ALUMINUM

Physical effects—Irritates intestines; affects bone formation and brain, dry mouth, dry stools, inhibits cell oxidation

Symptoms—Gastrointestinal irritation, colic, rickets, convulsions

Environmental sources—Aluminum cooking utensils, antacids, foils, deodorants, aluminum sulfate baking powders, processed foods containing aluminum, soft water

Protective nutrients—Vitamins E and C; herbal combination of pumpkin seed, okra, rhubarb root, capsicum, peppermint, and dulse

ARSENIC

Physical effects—Inhibits metabolism (reduces energy production efficiency), poisons cells and enzymes

Symptoms—Fatigue, low vitality, listlessness, loss of pain sensation, loss of body hair, skin color changes, dark spots, gastroenteritis, back pain

Environmental sources—Coal burning, pesticides, insecticides, herbicides, defoliants, metal smelting, cigarette smoke, manufacture of glass, mirrors

Protective nutrients—Iodine, selenium, sulfur, amino acids, vitamin C

CADMIUM

Physical effects—Heart and blood vessel structure (hypertension), kidneys, blocks appetite and smell centers, calcium metabolism, removes calcium from bones

Symptoms—Hypertension, kidney damage, loss of sense of smell, decreased appetite

Environmental sources—Cigarette smoke, oxide dusts, contaminated drinking water, galvanized pipes, paints, welding, pigments, contaminated shellfish from industrial seashores

Protective nutrients—Zinc, calcium, sulfur, amino acids, vitamin C

LEAD

Physical effects—Poisons enzymes, blocks enzymes at cell level, osteoblast production, blood formation

Symptoms—Weakness, listlessness, fatigue, pallor, abdominal discomfort, constipation, hyperactive children

Environmental sources—Leaded gas, lead-based paint, newsprint and colored ads, hair dyes and rinses, dolomite, soft coal, leaded glass, pewter ware, pesticides, pencils, fertilizers, pottery, cosmetics, tobacco smoke, polluted air (average 35 mg./day in U.S., higher in industrial areas and some cities)

Protective nutrients—Sulfur, amino acids, vitamins C and E, calcium, iron

MERCURY

Physical effects—Destroys cells, blocks transport of sugars (energy at cell levels), increases permeability of potassium (convulsions)

Symptoms—Loss of appetite and weight, severe emotional disturbances, tremors, blood changes, inflammation of gums, chewing and swallowing difficulty, inability to feel pain

Environmental sources—Manufacture and delivery of petroleum products, fungicides, fluorescent lamps, cosmetics, hair dyes, barometers, thermometers, amalgams in dentistry, salt water fish caught in contaminated waters

Protective nutrients—Pectin, sulfur, amino acids, vitamin C, selenium

Fluorine Poisoning

In a January 1955 *National Fluoridation News* article, Dr. G. L. Waldbott states, "A peculiar disease is making its appearance throughout the land. When those affected seek medical advice, doctors who are not yet familiar with this disease are liable to call them neurotics; they may even ridicule them. It is the initial stage of chronic fluorine poisoning."

As a rule, patients complain of the following symptoms:

- Irritation of the mouth from sores and ulcers
- Predisposition to upper respiratory
- Continuous backache along the spinal cord (spine becomes stiff
- Sharp, gnawing pains in the stomach, as though it were "burning inside"
- Nausea and loss of appetite
- The more water you drink, the more discomfort in the stomach
- Mental alertness deteriorates (can't think clearly)
- Numbness and weakness in the legs and arms, especially in the fourth and fifth fingers

- Unsteady feeling (sometimes legs give way; may fall down)
- Skin shows dry eruptions (seborrhea) on the chest

Dr. Leo Spira, who conducted experiments with fluorine on rats for four years, drew the following conclusions.

- Fluorine interferes with the proper utilization of vitamin B.
- Much damage is done to the kidneys, causing Bright's disease.
- The thyroid gland is greatly damaged by the action of fluorine.
- Fluorine causes the heart muscles to become flabby and degenerated.

The 1983 United States Pharmacoepia Volumes on Drug Information indicate that the following symptoms can appear in people taking tablets containing one-half to one milligram of fluoride per day (the amount of fluoride found in one to two pints of fluoridated water). Here are the symptoms:

- Black, tarry stools
- Bloody vomit
- Faintness
- Shallow breathing
- Tremors
- Watery eyes
- Weakness
- Loss of appetite
- Skin rash
- Stiffness
- Diarrhea
- Nausea and vomiting
- Stomach cramps or pain
- Unusual excitement
- Unusual increase in saliva
- Constipation
- Pain and aching of bones
- Sores in the mouth and on the lips

Fluoride Constitution

In his book, *Fluoride: The Aging Factor*, Dr. John Yiamouyiannis draws the following conclusions.

- Fluoride disturbs the chromosome repair enzyme.
- Sodium fluoride damages the immune system by weakening it as an old body is weakened (old-age problem).

- Sodium fluoride interrupts the amino acid chain in collagen.
- Fluoride dramatically slows the thought processes.

Fluoride is used to calm rioting prisoners. Fluoride does not have a discernable taste, not even in toothpaste. So much fluoride is added to one tube of toothpaste that a child could die from eating it.

Many years ago, when kidney dialysis machines were seldom used, Denver had one of the first centers. A physician from Houston, Texas, lived with us for a while, and he had a treatment every other day. He was so miserable, so sick, so disappointed, so down, that the only way to comfort him was by stroking his tortured body lightly, barely touching him.

One day I told him that the trouble was fluoride poisoning. He sat up in bed, his eyes widened. "Now I see the connection," he said.

"I wanted to have fluoride in the drinking water in Texas. In order to demonstrate the safeness of it, I drank a full glass of much fluoride-concentrated water. Nothing happened, but…a few days later, I had pain in the kidneys. I never connected it with that brave deed. Please help me to get it out of my kidneys," he said. I prayed for hours for this man, but he could not be saved.

The following information is taken from the book *Introduction to Biochemical Toxicology* by Ernest Hodgson and Frank Guthrie:

> Fluoride inhibits glycolysis but has no effect on oxygen consumption. Pronounced hyperglycemia and glycosuria are induced in rabbits by sodium fluoride. The hyperglycemia is reversible by insulin. Fluoride ion inhibits cholinesterase and several phosphatases and interferes with the metabolization of arginine and glutamine. Fluoroacetate is a metabolic poison by virtue of its strong inhibition of the tricarboxylic acid cycle. Fluoroacetate combines with oxaloacetic acid to form fluorocitric acid, which blocks tricarboxylic acid cycle activity and causes citric acid to accumulate in the tissues.

Sodium Fluoride

Sodium fluoride destroys our will to live. It settles in the neck on the left side and in the tissue, and it causes apathy; people become mentally lethargic. It promotes low blood sugar.

Since fluoride accumulates in the kidneys, they need special attention. In an adult, through osmosis, the fluoride in toothpaste can offset the iodine in the thyroid and the calcium hormones in the parathyroid in such a manner that the glandular system suffers. Also, the sugar system becomes unstable.

Dr. Yiamouyiannis stated that fluoride interrupts the chain of amino acids in collagen.

Researchers from Harvard University and the National Institutes of Health knew in the 1960s that fluoride disrupted collagen synthesis. It was not until 1979 to 1981, however, that a new flurry of research activity in this area began.

Collagen is composed of amino acids linked together in a chain. However, collagen contains two additional amino acids—hydroxyproline and hydroxylysine—not found in other proteins. Thus, when collagen synthesis is interfered with or when collagen breaks down, the hydroxyproline and hydroxylysine levels in the blood and urine increase breakdown of the collagen protein chain into its amino acid links. Thus, the high levels of the "free" hydroxyproline and hydroxylysine "links" induced by fluoride are conclusive evidence that fluoride is accelerating the breakdown of collagen.

What to Do

We have two distinct formulas to help. In lengthy laboratory experiments, it was found that manganese reduces the toxic effect of sodium fluoride considerably—so much so that manganese is now used widely all over the country.

Another big help is a tasty tea made from calendula, dandelion leaves, elder, nettle, red root, St. John's wort, and yarrow.

Sodium fluoride reduces the effectiveness of lactobacillus acidophilus that forms cariogenic lactic acid. This acid is needed to manufacture interferon, which is important in fighting cancer.

Cottage cheese mixed with raw oils aids the body's production of interferon. See Interferon, in chapter 6.

Plutonium

Raw plutonium stones are not harmful. They only become harmful when they are tampered with, isolated, or split. When it enters the air, plutonium explodes into three parts over one and a half days. Two of the parts are positively charged. They get into our bodies and cut the proteins, enzymes, and molecules into little pieces that float in the bloodstream and lymphatic system.

Radiation

Peat moss removes radiation, including x-rays, cancer, radiation cobalt, and fallout. A four- to six-inch bed of peat moss removes all radiation from the body in one night. Fifty to 100 pound sacks of moss are sold like dirt. It can be put under the bed or in flowerpots, and it is good for half a year under or around the television. Willow leaves are another radiation antidote. Miso, which is fermented bean paste, will protect you from radiation. Don't boil it.

In Hiroshima, after the A-bomb, people ate tomatoes and cucumbers for three months to clear the fallout from their systems.

Pesticides

Most pesticides are stored in the fatty deposits of the human body. If you go on a fat-reducing diet, these pesticides can bring on heart attack and/or severe nervous disorder. Therefore, take it easy with reducing diets.

Irradiated Food

The controversy grows. The use of the pesticide EDB on grains and fruits was banned because the chemical was found to cause cancer in animals, but the Food and Drug Administration (FDA) has proposed a possible alternative. The agency wants to allow the use of ionizing radiation—such as that emitted by x-ray machines—to kill pests on fruits, vegetables, and spices.

Now the question being asked is: Will acceptance of the proposal simply substitute one problem for another?

The FDA says no, based on 30 years of governmentally funded studies. It maintains that food irradiation is safe when used at doses not exceeding 100 kilorads. (A rad is a unit used to express an amount of absorbed radiation.) The agency claims that the process leaves no detectable radioactive residue on food and does not significantly reduce nutritional content. In addition, it can extend the shelf life of certain foods, such as potatoes and oranges, by inhibiting sprouting or ripening. But opponents of food irradiation argue that the safety of the process has not been firmly proven.

Radiation causes chemical changes that produce new substances in food. The FDA asserts that the changes are negligible. But some public interest groups, such as the Health and Energy Institute, and several scientists counter that there have not been enough long-term studies to support this claim. Further, they say, there is some evidence that irradiation increases the production of a naturally occurring carcinogen called aflatoxin.

What makes matters worse, critics charge, is that the FDA proposal does not recommend that irradiated food be labeled as such at the retail level. Some comments on the proposal suggest the public might believe food so labeled to be radioactive. But Kitty Tucker, Executive Director of the Health and Energy Institute, argues that "this amounts to protecting consumers by keeping them ignorant."

The FDA says the question of labeling is still open and that it might reword the proposal. But a decision will not be made until the agency has had a chance to review all of the nearly 4,000 public comments it has received on the plan.

Just how should food be irradiated? The Department of Energy (DOE) is pushing for a process that exposes food on a conveyer belt to pellets of cesium 137, a radioactive waste that can be generated from spent nuclear fuel. Tucker sees this as "a government attempt to turn garbage into gold." It would be safer, she says, to use particle accelerators or x-ray machines as sources of radiation. Unlike cesium 137, neither one needs to be transported on public highways, reducing the chance of accidental radioactive contamination.

Soma Board

Can't we detoxify our food, our juices, and our milk from heavy metal and chemical poisons before we put them on the table? Yes, we can! It was mothers who invented this gift to a nation in trouble.

Dr. Parcells developed the Magnetic Lamp. You put all food under it, and through magnetic energy, it offsets harmful chemicals.

I developed the Soma Board. It works like pyramid energy through transmutation of harmful elements. The two instruments in it, the blue transparent film and the herb-mineral mixture, perform the miracle.

The Soma Board is designed to bring more healthful vibrations into your kitchen. Almost all of our foods contain some chemicals, additives, or preservatives. These stay in your fruit or vegetables even when you wash all produce. Over the years, these additives accumulate, and allergic reaction sets in. The liver just cannot neutralize so much poison.

We have to do something about the additives in order to have healthy families. We have to neutralize these foreign substances that are in our food, fruit, and vegetables. Otherwise, we fall into a pattern of poor health.

Soma is built on the idea of pyramid energy. There is no pyramid inside the box, but just as the pyramid energy neutralizes chemicals, so does this invention neutralize poisons and chemicals. Soma is a unique combination of minerals and herbs that achieve the ionization of your food. By doing so, chemicals and metals are ionized and will be rendered harmless.

The Soma treatment makes everything taste better. The fruit tastes sweeter, bread tastes fabulous, water is milder, and so on. Even cigarettes change taste, making it easier to quit the habit. I take my Soma Board on air flights, and it neutralizes my food. Since I started using it, I don't come home with stomachaches anymore.

Chemical Additives in Your Food

Chemical additive: Red dye #2—Colors foods red, brown, purple, and
orange
Foods—Soft drinks, ice cream, cherries, candy, cake frostings
Health risk—Has produced tumors in test animals; only the United States,
Mexico, and Denmark permit this additive

Chemical additive: Yellow dye #5—Used to give gold-yellow color to foods
Foods—Beverages, desserts, candy, cereals, ice cream, baked goods, snack foods; also used in prescription drugs, pain relievers, and antihistamines
Health risk—Can cause allergic reactions, including wheezing, asthmatic symptoms, and hives

Chemical additive: Blue dye #1—Used to give a bluish color to foods
Foods—Soft drinks, gelatin desserts, ice cream, ices, dry drink powders, candy, cereals, puddings, bakery products
Health risk—May cause allergic reactions; tests show that it produces malignant tumors in animals

Chemical additive: BHA (butylated hydroxyanisole)—Prevents fats and oils from turning rancid
Foods—Cake mixes, shortenings, potato chips, breakfast cereals, gelatin desserts, candy, pudding and pie filling mixes, bakery products
Health risk—Can cause allergic reactions

Chemical additive: BHT (butylated hydroxytoluene)—Prevents fats and oils from turning rancid
Foods—Potato flakes, enriched rice, shortenings containing animal fats, frozen pork sausages, freeze-dried meats
Health risk—Can cause allergic reactions; tests have produced chemical changes in the brains of animal offspring; England prohibits its use in foods

Chemical additive: Glycerides—Emulsifies; defoaming agent
Foods—Bakery products, ice cream, ice milk, lard, chewing gum, shortenings, oleomargarine, sweet chocolate, whipped toppings
Health risk—Suspected to cause reproductive problems and malformations

Chemical additive: MSG (monosodium glutamate)—Used to enhance the flavor of foods
Foods—Canned and frozen foods, prepared meats, pickles, soups, candy, baked goods, mayonnaise, Accent (is mostly MSG); large amounts of this ingredient are used in many Chinese foods
Health risk—Affects nerve endings and can cause dizziness, numbness, headaches, and other symptoms

Chemical additive: Nitrites and nitrates (potassium and sodium)—Used as a color fixative in cured meats

Foods—Bacon, bologna, frankfurters, meat spreads, pickling brine, chopped meat, smoked ham, potted meats, poultry, smoked fish (including tuna, salmon, and shad); some meat tenderizers are almost 100 percent sodium nitrate (fertilizer)

Health risk—Combines with other substances to produce cancerous agents called nitrosamines and nitrosamides; can cause death by cutting off oxygen to the brain and heart

Chemical additive: Sulfur dioxide—Prevents dried fruits from fermenting and other foods from spoiling

Foods—Wines, corn syrup, dried fruits, dehydrated potatoes, soups, condiments

Health risk—Tends to deplete the body's supply of vitamin A; inhalation can produce respiratory irritation

Tumors

Abnormal growths take many forms. The most common types are described by physicians as cysts or tumors. Tumors can be either benign (noncancerous) or malignant (cancerous). Each kind of growth suggests different kinds of imbalances in a person's chemistry. Some people are predisposed to tumor formation because of these biochemical imbalances. People with similar problems often have significant differences in their chemistry.

Calcium

Calcium is extremely important in detoxifying environmental poisons in the body. Scientists have provided the following interesting facts. A living cell needs 10,000 enzymes to function properly. To detoxify this gigantic laboratory, it needs calcium. Without a proper calcium supply, the enzymes cannot be utilized.

Calcium also deactivates radioactive substances. It is known that radioactive material lodges in the brain easily. A proper supply of calcium protects us and screens off the foreign substances.

An interesting book, *Nuclear Medicine*, by Dr. H. Sack and Dr. G. Legmann, suggests the importance of calcium in nuclear exposure, x-rays, and other ray exposures.

It has also been suggested that we increase our vitamin E intake. Vitamin E is capable of neutralizing and binding carbon monoxide, carbon dioxide, and environmental pollution from car exhaust.

Karma

The spiritual side to chemical and metallic poison is karma. Karmic conditions are rare, but they do exist. It is one of the seven spiritual causes of ill health. Karma is unfinished business. If your illness is of karmic nature, you need to work twice as hard to overcome this unfinished business.

Energy follows thought. This is one of the laws of the universe, and we have to keep this in mind. If we have happy and constructive thoughts, energy will follow these kinds of thoughts and build a healthy environment and a healthy body. If we have thoughts of jealousy, hate, destruction, envy, and fear, we are inviting energies of the darkness. I don't mean necessarily illness, but an environment in which difficulties of an inner nature will appear and hinder the work you came to do in this lifetime. If you are slowed down, frustrated in reaching your goal, and unable to express yourself creatively, you become ill.

Creative expression is the most important factor in staying well.

❧ CHAPTER FIVE ❧

Worms and Parasites As a Cause of Ill Health

When metals, chemicals, pesticides, and environmental poisons cannot be neutralized by the liver and every function of the body goes down, then worms set in. Worms are scavengers. If a plant lacks healthy soil, parasites will destroy what is left of its sickly frame. It is the same with us—if our body chemistry is down, all kinds of worms and parasites can and will move in.

Good health starts with cleaning out the waste, including worms and parasites.

Worms and parasites are powerful contributors to ill health. It is important to recognize pinworms, roundworms, tapeworms, and the much feared dog tapeworm. It is also necessary to get acquainted with parasites from foreign countries. Scientists know of about 120 different kinds of parasites that can and do invade the human body.

Where Do Worms Come From?

Imagine an uncovered cup of vinegar on your counter. The vinegar is swarming with tiny flies. Take the vinegar away, and all of the flies vanish. Where did they come from? Where did they go? No one knows.

Worms also need a medium to live in, just as vinegar flies need vinegar. Worms need one of the following environments to survive:

- A toxic colon
- Chemicals or other poisons
- An alkaline medium

Let's go back to the vinegar on your countertop. If we clean up the breeding place, the flies disappear. If we clean up the bloodstream's environmental poisons, there is nothing for the scavengers to live on. One gallon of hyssop tea daily for two days is a terrific cleansing method for the body's toxic condition.

Worms and parasites disturb the balance of the entire system. Worms can cause the following problems:

- Mineral imbalance
- Loss of sleep
- Thyroid imbalances
- Blood in stool
- Allergies such as asthma
- Pain all over the body
- High blood sugar (e.g., diabetes)

- Loss of hair
- Headaches
- Intestinal gas
- Chronic prostatitis
- Eczema
- Arthritis

How to Recognize Worms

An iridologist can discover parasites early, but when people have coal black eyes, even an iridologist is out of luck. Iridology is a carried-down science of the blue-eyed races. It was used over centuries, and it is still in use where blue-eyed races are the majority. Native Americans, however, looked at the soles of the feet and in the grooves, marks, and blemishes discovered mankind's biggest enemy—parasites.

Parasites take on the vibration of their host; therefore, they are difficult to detect. I don't think it is as much what these creatures eat that is damaging to the human body, but that their waste is extremely poisonous to us. A healthier environment throughout the body is needed to discourage the existence of these scavengers and their breeding places.

If a person is very nervous at the full moon, he may have worms and/or parasites. Tapeworms create a high sugar level in the blood. When there is sugar increase in the urine, ask your physician for a tapeworm examination.

Any treatment for worms should be done during the full moon. Tapeworms and roundworms are moon animals. They sleep a great deal of the moon cycle. They wake up, multiply, and become obnoxious around the full moon. That's when the laboratory technician can find them. The following indications alert you to the presence of worms and parasites:

- Pyloric valve trouble (indicates worms in the liver)
- Nervousness around the full moon
- Five- to seven-pound weight gain around the full moon
- Grinding teeth at night (watch for in children)

Worms and parasites take the best of your blood and leave their waste, which is poisonous. They eat your vitamins, and the more vitamins you take, the worse you feel. Worms do not like minerals.

Tapeworm

When rolled up, tapeworms create a ball under the ribs on the right side below the liver. Sometimes this ball is there; sometimes it is gone. Sometimes there is an increase of weight up to seven pounds around the full moon; constipation and diarrhea alternate; and some people lose weight. However, most people are overweight when afflicted with this problem. A tiny tapeworm has been discovered in household cats that presents a potential threat to human health. If transferred from cats to humans, this parasite can affect the liver, lungs, and brain.

Salmonella

What is salmonella? It is a tiny organism that likes to live in chicken and other meat products and eggs. In its mildest form, it is a nuisance. The FDA reports that 250,000 persons are hit annually by salmonella. People call it the 24-hour "bug." It causes nausea, fever, diarrhea, stomach cramps, and vomiting. In some cases, including children under the age of four, people who already have a weakened condition, or the elderly, salmonella symptoms can become dangerous. Other people become depressed, feverish, and miserable, and it can go on for years.

To prevent salmonella, the Department of Health and Human Sciences (HHS) warns us to wash with soap and hot water all dishes that were contaminated with raw meat during preparation of a meal. Wash hands after touching raw meat, and refrigerate all dairy and egg products.

Hookworm

The Latin name for hookworm is *Ancylostomatidae*. There is one kind that prefers to live on the duodenum. Hookworms are small—only half a centimeter long or smaller—but by sucking blood they are dangerous.

No human worm infection has attracted so much attention and has been the subject of so much investigation as hookworm. This is justifiable, for no other worm infection is as significant to the human race as a whole. Hookworm is never as spectacular as other diseases, but it is insidious. Year after year, generation after generation, it sucks the vitality and undermines the health and efficiency of whole communities. In the course of a few summers, a healthy family may become pale and puny. Once industrious, they become languid and backward. Once prosperous, they fall into debt. Once proud, property-owning people, they are reduced to tenancy and poverty. The children, once bright and intelligent, become dull and indifferent and soon fall hopelessly behind in school and drop out.

Toxoplasmosis

Toxoplasmosis was a medical mystery until just recently. Dr. Dean Jacobs, assistant director of collaborative research for the National Institute of Health, explained that at least 500 million people throughout the world are infected with toxoplasmosis. The parasite that caused this disease is so small that 1,000 of them can exist on a speck of dirt as small as half a dime.

Dr. B. H. Kean, chemical professor of tropical medicine at Cornell University in New York, says, "We know that any rare meat could cause the infection (toxo), and now we know that cats can spread toxoplasmosis, too. Cats who have toxo spread it through their waste to anyone handling the waste." Dr. Kean and other experts estimate that 78 million people in the United States are infected with toxoplasmosis. The infection may lie dormant for many years only to break out when resistance is low.

Dr. Jacob Karl Trankel, professor of pathology at the University of Kansas Medical School, says, "There are people who have contracted toxoplasmosis and were unscathed, but the infection lies dormant in them. An attack of the dormant parasites may be triggered when sick people are given immune suppressive drugs, to fight foreign invaders, so that the parasites suddenly begin multiplying."

Toxoplasmosis has been mistaken for other diseases for many years because so little was known about it. The effects of toxoplasmosis can resemble the following illnesses:

- Mononucleosis
- Anemia
- Low blood sugar
- Hodgkin's disease
- Heart attack
- Pneumonia
- Leukemia
- Brain tumors
- Blindness

Toxoplasmosis is critically dangerous to newborn babies, as Dr. Leo Yercalis notes. A child whose mother has the infection during pregnancy has only one chance in two of escaping this disease, which may cause mental illness, deformities, and brain damage.

Eighty-six percent of low blood sugar cases have toxoplasmosis.

Dr. Calbert Phillips, from Royal Eye Hospital in England, writes: "Toxocara worm is a cat worm that can cause eye diseases when children or adults accidentally swallow the tiny eggs. Fever, convulsions, enlarged liver and spleen may also be caused by Toxocara worm."

Trichinosis

Trichinosis is the name of a medically "incurable" disease in swine and humans. It is caused by a parasite, Trichinella spiralis (trichina), and was discovered by James Paget in 1835. Encysted, it is found in human muscle, including the heart. Not until 1846 was trichina located as a source of trouble in swine. By 1859, scientist Rudolph Leuchart had documented the entire cycle of the trichina in humans.

It is impossible to accurately estimate how many millions of human beings are infected with trichina and probably treated and overtreated for diseases they do not have. According to the 1962 edition of the *Encyclopedia Britannica*, it is estimated that some 28 million people throughout the world are infected, with 21 million (75 percent) of the victims being in the United States.

The United States Department of Agriculture (USDA) provides for no inspection of pork and other meat products for the presence of trichina on the basis that it would cost too much, because there is no method known for discovering the parasite other than microscopic examination. The only attempted protection is the requirement that such pork-containing products as wieners, salami, and so forth are cooked.

Symptoms include weakness, fatigue, headache, sore throat, chills and fever with sweating, laryngitis with cough, and swelling around the eyes and face. Often there is a rash present on the trunk or upper extremities, and/or fluid retention. Statistically, it is reported that 40 percent of all lung cancer and brain cancer have their origins in the weakening of these organs by trichinosis.

Trichinosis is a disease that has been completely wiped out in Europe and other countries. How did Europe wipe out trichinosis? Trichinosis is a disease of swine. No other animal carries it. Around 1903, the health departments of all European countries met and discussed the possibility of wiping out the feared trichinosis poisoning through pork.

Germany was the instigator. Every hog that came to the market for meat was examined. A piece of the brain was removed. When there was trichinosis present, the state bought the hog at full market price so that the farmer did not lose anything. Then the state had all the farmers' hog sheds cleaned out. Eventually, this disease was wiped out, and now pork is safe to eat in Europe. There was a small flare-up after World War II when uninspected pork from foreign countries hit the markets. For a time, swine and all other animals were checked for trichinosis again.

Trichinosis hits the brain of the animal first, then the lungs, then the muscles. Trichinosis-infected animals either run in circles or are prone to heart attack; therefore, they are sold very young in the United States before these symptoms have a chance to appear.

Protozoa

Dr. Roger Wyburn-Mason, British medical specialist at Ealing and Houndslow Holp in West London, claims to have found both the cause and cure for rheumatoid arthritis, one of the world's most crippling diseases. He is convinced that the disease is the result of protozoan infections. Protozoa are minute, one-celled animals that live as parasites in the bloodstream.

Dr. Bingham, M.D., in his famous book, *Fight Back Against Arthritis*, wrote: "The presence of protozoa in the tissue can be the cause of continual inflammation in people who are genetically or otherwise sensitive to the organism."

Protozoa can cause other degenerative diseases, including the following:

- Paget's disease of the bones
- Myasthenia gravis
- Chronic nephritis
- Some cases of pericarditis
- Some cases of lymphoma
- Some cases of leukemia
- Scleroderma
- Melanoderma
- Psoriasis
- Asthma
- Ulcerative colitis
- Arthritis
- Some cases of diabetes
- Some cases of hepatitis
- Some cases of Hodgkin's disease
- Some cases of ovarian cysts
- Vitiligo
- Eczema
- Pyorrhea
- Chronic bronchitis
- Parkinson's disease of the central nervous system

The blood of healthy people contains antibodies against these organisms.

Parasite/Worm Remedies

Tapeworm—Use an herbal combination of pumpkin seed, garlic, cramp bark, capsicum, and thyme. Eat plenty of pumpkin seeds in all cases of worms. Weight problems and sugar imbalance are often seen with tapeworm trouble.

Roundworm—*First option:* Use an herbal combination of black walnut leaves, wormwood, quassia, cloves, and male fern.

Second option: Give as much garlic as patient can stand; two days later give a laxative. Have the patient sit in a milk bath sufficient for covering the rectal area. Worms smell the milk and crawl out. Keep patient in the warm bath for about one hour until all the worms are out. This can be rather unpleasant.

Third option: Eat Calimyrna figs to make intestine uninhabitable by roundworms.

Blood fluke, ascaris, and others—Pumpkin seeds are the best natural remedy.

Use this recipe: Grate an apple, add pumpkin seeds, and top with yogurt. A fine breakfast for children and adults.

Salmonella—*First option:* Try homeopathic *Ipecacuanha*, or ipecac syrup; take eight drops in water every hour, four hours in a row, for three weeks.

Second option: Try a homeopathic remedy specific to salmonella.

Third option: Use an herbal combination of echinacea, black walnut leaves, and Russian black radish. Grind to powder, fill in capsules. Take two capsules three times daily before meals.

Pinworms—Take two cloves of garlic, mash them thoroughly, boil in six ounces of milk, let cool, and strain. Prepare an enema: Inject four ounces of this milk into rectum. Do this for three nights in a row. Wait seven days and repeat.

Blood parasite (reportedly found in all cancer cases)—Combine equal parts of oil of sassafras, wintergreen, and spruce. Mix and rub four drops on the soles of the feet three times daily.

Hookworm—During WWI, hookworms were treated with thymol and chenopodium oil. Now, a nontoxic solution comes from England—a homeopathic remedy specific to hookworm.

Anaplasmosis (tick fever)—Combine chaparral tea and two drops of anise oil; drink twice daily. Also use thyme oil and pine oil externally.

Toxoplasmosis—Mix sassafras oil and pine oil in equal parts. Rub three drops on the soles of the feet two times daily.

Trichinosis—Take three drops of wintergreen oil in one teaspoon of molasses twice daily for three months. After three months, take three magnesium oxide tablets twice daily for three weeks.

Protozoa—Eliminate the following foods: white potatoes, eggplant, tomatoes, and red peppers. Before each meal, take three tablets homeopathic *Cuprum metallicum*, three tablets homeopathic *Ipecacuanha*, and ten drops of a homeopathic specific to protozoa.

All varieties—Use this recipe: two capsules wormwood, one capsule sage, and three capsules capsicum, twice daily for 15 days.

Worms in bladder—Combine black walnut, sassafras, and pine needles.

Worms in tissue—Combine male fern, yellow dock, black walnut, and cloves.

Spiritual Scavengers and Invaders

As parasites and worms can hurt, injure, and cause great damage to the human body, so may possession, obsessions, voodoos, curses, and black magic cause considerable damage to our bodies and to our lives. To protect yourself, stay in the light, pray over your children, pray over your food, and send messages of love and waves of joy. Help each other, and know that you are never alone.

Spastic Entities and Ailments

One of the principal effects of invading or possessing entities is that they introduce spastic complaints. Entities comprise an integral part of the causation of epilepsy, spastic paralysis, cerebral palsy, etc. They are involved in some cases of high blood pressure from hypertension. They sometimes play a part in asthma. All individuals suffering from any type of spastic symptoms should be tested thoroughly for the entire factor. Occasionally one will see an individual who suffers from voice shutoffs. He or she will be talking, and suddenly there is an inability to get the sound out. The voice muscles in the larynx have gone spastic—invariably through the interference of entities.

Obsession in Blood Caused by Transfusions

The only published reference to this subject that I have found thus far occurs in the book *Homeopathy for the First-Aider*, by Dr. Dorothy Shepherd, published by Health Science Press of England. Dr. Shepherd found that electronic tunings for obsession registered in the blood of individuals who had received transfusions or had given blood to others, while individuals who had never given or received blood practically never exhibited any obsession in the bloodstream. Treating the obsession out of the bloodstream brought about a marked improvement in the physical and emotional welfare of the patient.

She states that "blood, as the vehicle of life, is specific to each individual, containing properties peculiar to each person; aggravations and conflicts, physical, mental, and spiritual, are likely to ensue when foreign blood is introduced. We know not what the ultimate outcome will be, a total change of personality is likely....This is too long and serious a subject to be dealt with in a few short phrases."

The vibratory disharmony created by blood transfusions creates an attraction for obsessing entities, just as a diseased condition attracts entities. When this disharmony is in the bloodstream, the invading entities associate themselves with the blood, creating the particular condition designated by the author as obsession of the blood.

What to Do

The Ray method, introduced by Dr. John Ray, is used to remove subtle invasions of the body. Dr. Ray's main work and his terrific results stem from the fact that spastic entities can be released by holding certain trigger points on the body. It is a fascinating work.

Before you start Dr. Ray's method, be sure to get a pulsor. A pulsor is a protective device that guards your aura against released invaders. Be sure that you pray, and don't let go even if it takes hours of release work. The sternal notch seems to be the main release point.

Dr. Ray's work is very welcome, because few churches take time to remove entities from their faithful and trusting parishioners. Jesus said, "Heal the sick and rebuke the dark forces."

Prayer Action Plan

The Hawaiian Kahunas used to get rid of unwanted negative attitudes and feelings by relaxing and commanding those unwanted negative attitudes to leave their bodies as they shook their right and left legs.

Here is another suggestion for maintaining spiritual well-being.

1. Review the situation that is presently causing a particular emotional stress.
2. Pick a word that expresses the positive opposite of this negative emotion (for example, hate ➤ love; anxiety ➤ security; worry ➤ confidence; impatience ➤ patience; etc.).
3. Place a glass of water next to you.
4. Relax. See yourself beset with negative emotion. Put it all into the glass of water. Throw the water away.
5. Take a fresh cup, preferably porcelain. Fill this cup with water and think that this water contains the necessary solution to your problem—it is filled with the opposite, positive emotion. Drink the water, knowing you are filling yourself with the positive emotion you need, and the negativity will leave you when you next urinate.
6. End session. Then urinate, feeling an exhilaration of positivity.

The Healing Magic of Crystals

The most outstanding authority on crystal powers is Marcel Vogel, a senior scientist with IBM for 27 years until his retirement in early 1984. He says, "At first this may sound paradoxical, but there are no powers whatsoever in the crystal. The crystal is a neutral object whose inner structure exhibits a state of perfection and balance. When it's cut to the proper form and when the human mind enters into relationships with its structural perfection, the crystal emits a vibration that extends and amplifies the powers of the user's mind. Like a laser, it radiates energy in a coherent, highly concentrated form, and this energy may be transmitted into objects or people at will.

"As psychics have often pointed out, when a person becomes emotionally distressed, a weakness forms in his subtle energy body and disease may soon follow. With a properly cut crystal, however, a healer can—like a surgeon cutting away a tumor—release negative patterns of energy in the body, allowing the physical body to return to a state of wholeness."

A crystal multiplies the thought-form and also holds the thought-form invoked in it. Therefore, a crystal always has to be cleansed before and after using it for healing or for entity removal. A crystal is a tool just as a pendulum or a dowsing rod is a tool; however, a crystal is a very delicate device. It is a tool for healing the etheric body. It is a tool for healing the aural body.

How do you clear and clean a crystal?

I know of the following four methods:

1. Soak crystal in salt water.
2. Place crystal on a violet-colored velvet cloth (which I have cut in the shape of a cross).
3. Blow at the crystal from all sides to release the thought-form.
4. Place the crystal in a dish of Hawaiian red salt (this is very powerful).

After clearing and cleansing the crystal, this tool is ready to be used.

How can you use a crystal?

The seat of our life-force energy is a point in the sternum two inches below the thymus gland. In fact, the entire sternum indicates the strength of each individual's life force. It is at this point, close to the thymus, where we have to contact the impaired life force and heal it with the crystal. It is the point of contact, the key to the etheric body of a Western man (the key for an Easterner is the solar plexus).

It was taught to me in the following manner: After clearing the crystal, I make 12 counterclockwise circles around the thymus gland, including the point two inches below the gland. Then I clear the crystal and make 12 clockwise circles over the same area. Then I hold the crystal between my eyes and command that the crystal will send the life force for healing wherever it is needed. I hold the crystal over the thymus and command again in the name of Jesus that the etheric body of the person will be healed. When the etheric body and the aura are healed, the physical body has to heal also.

When someone is burned or injured, do the same thing over the burn or injury. If someone is possessed, do it 12 times counterclockwise over the entire body. Blow the crystal over a candle flame and command the dark ones to go into the light. Then go over the body 12 times in a clockwise manner and close the energy field of the life-force at the sternum either with the cross or with the directed laser beam of the crystal. I do it with the words Jesus taught us: "Tali Tha Cumi"—"Thou shall be whole."

It was revealed, in newly discovered scrolls, that Jesus carried two crystals with him, one on the right side and one on the left side in the folds of his garment. Jesus gave us the words to release these foreign energies. He said; "Eph-pha-pha-open" and "Satan, go behind." Then he lifted up his head and gave thanks to his Father that it was done. And he taught this to his disciples and said: "This and more thou shall do in my name."

PEARLS FROM THE BIBLE FOR HEALING

Proverbs 17:22: *A merry heart doeth good like a medicine: but a broken spirit drieth the bones.*

Isaiah 38:21: *For Isaiah had said, Let them take a lump of figs, and lay it for a plaster upon the boil, and he shall recover.*

Proverbs 24:13: *My son, eat thou the honey, because it is good; and the honeycomb, which is sweet to thy taste.*

Ezekiel 16:6 (repeat three times): *And when I passed by thee, and saw thee polluted in thine own blood, I said unto thee when thou wast in thy blood, Live; yea, I said unto thee when thou wast in thy blood, Live.*
(If bleeding is present, it will stop.)

Three times in a row, three times daily, say, "By his stripes, thou shall be healed." You will be amazed what a relief this is to you when you have pain.

⇜ CHAPTER SIX ⇝

Infections As a Cause of Ill Health

Since the initial writing of this book, science has come up with 2,200 diseases. Their names are in Latin or Greek. Some have their origin in Sanskrit. Some come from the Hebrew language. Most of us cannot understand these languages, so we are in awe about the names of the diseases. In fact, some people come to me and say, "I have a neat, rare disease. Did you ever hear about this?" Then they take a long breath and say a long word in a secret language, and they are proud that they could say the word and proud that they have such a rare disease. When we look it up in the medical dictionary, it may be epilepsy of unknown origin or worms in the lung.

The secrecy of this language reminds me of the churches in the Middle Ages. After Martin Luther had translated the Bible, populations of this earth were freed from ignorance. I go with the words of Christ, "Know the truth, and the truth shall make you free."

Immune System

Your immune system is your body's powerful defense against infections of all kinds—bacteria, fungi, and viruses. As long as your immune system is working, none of these invaders can harm you.

As we know it now, the following organs contribute to the existence of this powerful, spiritual system:

- Thymus gland (the heart of your immune system)
- Spleen
- Thyroid

What really takes place at this point, no one knows. It is suggested that the thymus gland makes and controls T cells. T cells are certain white blood cells that attack bacteria, viruses, and other infection-causing elements.

It is said that T cells are the bosses of the lymphocytes and also bosses of the antibody molecules. Lymphocytes are called B cells. We have one trillion lymphocytes that are under the command of T cells. What a job!

As we get older, the immune system becomes less powerful, less able to throw off infections. Infections in elderly people are always serious, and it takes longer for them to recuperate once they have an infection.

The spleen is definitely a part of the immune system; yet when it has to be removed because of an accident, the immune system does not collapse. The thyroid, when properly functioning, makes thyroid hormones that stimulate the immune system. It gives spark, zest, and life to the immune system. When the thyroid is under the influence of poisons, this spark cannot be created. Once your immune system fails to protect you, you are in trouble. Bacteria, viruses, and fungi find ways to enter the bloodstream, lymphatic system, and cells.

Infections and diseases can be harmless or very serious. We are surrounded by bacteria, viruses, and fungus-causing diseases. We are surrounded by protozoa. We are surrounded by all kinds of diseases. Those diseases cannot harm us as long as our immune system is fit. Our immune system can be weakened by too little sleep, too much smoking, or too much alcohol; by chemicals, pesticides, metallic poisons, and protoplasmic poison; and by ELF (extremely low frequency) waves.

What Causes the Immune System to Break Down?

The immune system suffers under the influence of chemicals, pesticides, chemotherapy, Candida albicans, pulling food over the scanner, and radiation of all kinds (including the radiation of food for preservation).

The immune system seems to operate on an electromagnetic principle. If we supply enough specific herbs and special food supplements, we may be able to keep it working. The following are remedies that God sent for the immune system.

- Grind up chaparral, capsicum, goldenseal, and echinacea; fill capsules or use as an extract.

- Vitamin A has a stimulating effect on the immune system.

- Vitamin C foods are stimulating to spleen and thyroid.

- Manganese is necessary for the thymus gland, making it whole some and revitalizing the immune system.

- Make sure there is enough zinc in your diet. Zinc deficiency can cause shrinkage of the thymus gland.

- Digestive enzymes found in pineapple and papaya are good for your immune system.

- One of the most powerful plants to increase and balance the immune system is quaw bark, what I call the American Pau d'arco.

Quaw Bark

Alec de Montmorency, an expert in exotic medicines and folk remedies, reportedly discovered a tree in Brazil called Pau d'arco, or Lapacho. The Brazilian Indians used the inner bark of this tree in the treatment of various diseases, including tumors and cancer, with unique results.

Pau d'arco has a tremendously healing vibration for people born and living in the Southern Hemisphere where energy moves in a counter-clockwise pattern. People born and living in the Northern Hemisphere, where energies move in a clockwise vibration, respond less favorably to Brazilian Pau d'arco.

In my diligent search for a tree in the Northern Hemisphere that would provide special healing virtues, I consulted with the Sioux and Oglala Indians for enlightenment. They directed me to the tree they call the quoiase or quaw tree.

Quaw bark (what I call the American Pau d'arco) regenerates cells and improves the production of red blood corpuscles. These Indians use the inner bark of the tree, which they claim gives them strength, stamina, and endurance, and also builds up the immune system.

The Indians use this bark for toxemia, varicose veins, hemorrhoids, hemophilia, and tumors (including cancer). It strengthens the pituitary gland and tones the entire glandular system. They also use it to help complete the healing process of old wounds and to offset the damage done by acne. It is most beneficial when used for fungus infection of the nails, skin fungus, and psoriasis.

Quaw bark definitely increases life-force, which may further explain why the Indians use it for longevity.

Blood Cleanser

To cleanse the blood, take one gallon of hyssop tea sweetened with honey or maple syrup for two days in a row. No food is needed.

Interferon

Part of the immune system, interferon prevents viruses from penetrating body cells. In all fungus diseases, including cancer, the body lacks interferon. This protein was discovered and named in 1957. It is produced naturally in the body by white cells and fibroblasts, as a response to occurrences of viruses.

So far, the following three types of interferon have been isolated:

- Leukocyte interferon in white blood cells
- Fibroblast interferon in connective tissues
- Immune interferon, produced by the so-called T cells, originating in the thymus gland

Interferon appears to function primarily as an intracellular messenger. Once a cell under viral attack produces interferon, the protein migrates through the cell membrane, spreading to other cells not yet attacked and triggering the production of antiviral proteins that are believed to block or interfere with viral reproduction.

The body produces interferon in minute quantities. One milligram of interferon requires 65,000 pints of blood, and it is species specific. Animal interferon has been achieved; hence its administration as a drug is extremely expensive.

Use the following recipe to make your own interferon:

Interferon Recipe Foundation:
Put in blender or mix thoroughly by hand: One cup cottage cheese and two tablespoons walnut, almond, or apricot oil. This mixture is the foundation recipe and can be varied.

Variations:

- Add finely grated horseradish. Serve with potatoes or buckwheat and/or stewed carrots.
- Add spices, such as finely cut parsley, celery, or paprika.
- Add tomatoes or tomato puree to taste. This is very delicious with rice, bulgur, or rye bread.
- Sweeten with honey or serve as a salad dressing.

Interferon is not only a must to stay healthy, but according to Dr. Uchida, interferon is used as an anti-herpes agent. It offsets the herpes infection.

The immune system is the mother of the lymphatic system. Without the T cells of the immune system, the lymph cannot function.

Lymphatic System

The lymphatic system is extremely important. It has its own channels and disintegrates at death. When you have a hard, callous ring around your heel or foot, you have a lymph problem. The lymphatic system is pumped by movement. It does not work when you are at rest. Running and working out moves the lymphatic system. If there is little opportunity for outdoor activity, keep a small trampoline rebounder in the house. Just a few minutes' workout on a rebounder two or three times daily will activate the lymphatic system, which is vital for good health.

Our forefathers walked to work and were refreshed when they arrived because the lymphatic system had had a workout. We must have the same— a stimulant, a workout—for our lymphatic system.

What to Do

To help lymph congestion, try the following remedy: Start with five juniper berries a day. Chew them slowly between meals, twice daily. Every day, add a juniper berry so that you increase to 15 juniper berries two times daily. Then, every day, reduce the number by one until you are back to five, twice daily. Chew them one at a time. When there are 15 berries, it will take you close to an hour to chew so many.

Congestion in the lymphatic system is favorably influenced by this procedure.

Protein

You shouldn't eat any protein after 2 P.M. The lymphatic system is very sensitive to protein imbalance, amino acid imbalance, and what we call "locked protein." When you eat any kind of concentrated protein such as eggs, fish, meat, cheese, soy products, or fowl, it will take eight hours to break this protein down to amino acids—the building blocks of the cells.

The liver does this tremendous job. After eight hours, the amino acids are ready to leave the liver to do their work. The lymphatic system is the transportation system. If you are asleep, the lymphatic system is also at rest and has only a few "emergency lines" going. The building blocks—the new chains of amino acids—to repair your worn-out cells cannot reach the places needing repair, and they are locked somewhere, usually in a weak spot in your body. For example, if you have a tumor, amino acids will collect there. In the case of arthritis, amino acids collect in your already stiff and painful muscles. If you eat heavy protein at 6 P.M., you will feed your troubles. The cancer will grow big and fat, and you will starve yourself to death.

Cell Respiration

In a living cell, milk cyclone fermentation can have D-positive or D-negative aspects, in scientific terms. The prolonged left-turning cycle of D-negative milk fermentation causes cell deterioration. It stops cell respiration so that the cell nucleus forms its own entity.

Dr. Englehardt demonstrated that the heart muscle can only use D-positive milk cyclone for its electrochemical balance and strength. It is obvious that other muscles require the same for maintenance and repair. The skin is particularly benefited by D-positive foods. D-positive milk cyclone activates the lymphatic system and detoxifies the entire body from environmental and other poisons.

What can we do to improve our defense system? What can we do to assure that D-positive milk cyclone is formed? Many cultures and nations have their own national drink or food that in one way or another is served in a fermented state. For example, in Bulgaria, Iran, and Turkey, it is a daily drink—kefir—made from yogurt and thinned down with spring water. In Germany, it is sauerkraut; in Scandinavia, raw fish; in South America there is a fermented drink; and on and on.

We can all have such benefits, but since we lack knowledge, very few of us use a fermented food or drink every day.

Beets are some of the richest D-positive foods—red beets are best of all. Just one teaspoon of beet powder will suffice. A soup with red beets or relish made out of beets will turn the cell to D-positive. Beets are also a detoxifier of environmental poisons.

In the past, we had thought that the color in beets is what prevents metastasis of cancer, but through the biochemical and electrobiochemical work of researchers, we find that it is the positive influences of beets on the D-negative cell that makes the miracles.

True prayers can turn the D-negative, biochemical, electrochemical stream into D-positive expression, and instant healing will result.

Apple whey is also beneficial. Combine one quart water, one quart apple juice, and one quart milk. Bring to a boil. As soon as it curdles, strain through a sieve. Drink very little at first—six ounces twice daily. Then increase the quantity to one quart daily. The lymph will respond, and the environmental toxins will be neutralized.

Bacterial Infections

Half of all the antibiotics used in the United States are fed to farm animals. A study in the *New England Journal of Medicine* reported that this has led to the growth of drug-resistant bacteria that are harmful to humans. The study is the first evidence that bacteria are attacking humans after evolving inside farm creatures to become immune to common antibiotics. These drug-resistant genes pass from one kind of bacteria to another, and doctors warn that they may make other common disease-causing germs hard to kill with currently available drugs.

Doctors believe that people acquire bacteria with these genes by eating animal products such as beef or milk. In this country, farmers routinely feed antibiotics to cows, hogs, and other animals to prevent disease and promote growth.

Strep Infections

Thank God we have penicillin, tetracycline, and other antibiotics. The fact that we do not understand how to take proper care after using penicillin is our own shortcoming. Penicillin is a mold, a fungus. It is superior in nature to strep infection, and more powerful; therefore, it is used to combat it. However, the side effect is obvious. We have to take care of the side effect—the fungus. Otherwise, we throw out Satan in exchange for Beelzebub.

When penicillin is needed, follow doctor's orders, but take care of the aftereffects. Penicillin kills all bacteria—friendly and unfriendly—and one has to fill the void created. I suggest you do this methodically and intelligently. After you take your last penicillin pill, start taking acidophilus. Buy seven bottles of liquid acidophilus and take half a bottle every day for 14 days. If you do not like the taste of acidophilus, buy some in capsules, and take three capsules before each meal for at least 14 days.

A bacterium cannot enter a living cell. It will surround the cell and multiply in the waste it creates. Therefore, large doses of vitamin C do an excellent job by clearing the waste surrounding the cell; then the bacteria die. Penicillin and derivatives are useful because the fungus kills the intruding bacteria but does not injure the cell. Bacterial infection can produce heart failure; therefore, consult your physician.

For those who cannot take penicillin, here are some time-proven natural remedies.

- Take 1,000 mg. vitamin C every hour for 10 hours when bacterial infection strikes.
- Take large doses of vitamin A in the same dose at the same time the first and second day.

- Crush the pit of an avocado. Boil in one pint water and take several tablespoons every hour (very effective against strep infection).

- For strep infection: Grate cucumber and squeeze the juice out. Drink five ounces five times daily.

- For infection in lungs: Boil onions, mash, and place between two layers of cloth. Apply to chest for about two hours. Repeat if needed.

- Use compresses of warm milk all over the body. Wrap patient in three layers—a warm milk sheet, a woolen blanket, and a warm cover. In two hours, repeat if needed. Bacteria like milk better than blood.

- Take an herbal combination of black radish root and parsley leaves. This is very effective if someone cannot take penicillin.

- Make tea from linden and elderberry.

- Use garlic against strep. Garlic's botanical name is *Allium sativum*. The use of garlic can be traced back as far as Babylonian times. The Chinese used garlic, and so did the Egyptians and the Romans. Garlic contains the antibacterial substance allicin. It is so powerful that it is used in the battle against gram-positive and gram-negative bacteria with satisfying results.

  If your physician permits you to try garlic for strep throat, use it with sage tea. Combine one heaping tablespoon sage to one quart of boiling water. Steep it for five minutes and remove from heat. Add one tablespoon garlic juice to the quart of sage tea. Gargle with it every two hours, and also drink four to six ounces several times daily.

Staph Infections

This takes a particular place in all types of infectious diseases. Staph is difficult to get rid of once you have it. The following symptoms appear:

- Listlessness
- Temperatures come and go
- Feelings of being lost
- Spells of despair
- Wounds heal slowly
- Boils break up, always blue afterward

- Acne-type boils on back or other places, always blue afterward

Staph infection can hide for a long time, only to break out in stressful situations. You need to go to a physician. Also, find out about oxyquinoline sulfate. This is derived from the nontoxic part of the cinchona tree whose bark yields quinine. It is a big help in the battle against staph infection.

Herpes II is a form of staph combined with a virus. Take all the suggestions of your physician and add oxyquinoline sulfate. Also, grate the skin of a grapefruit on a fine grater. Take one teaspoon and add the juice of one-half a grapefruit. Drink this three times daily.

Viral Infections

There is no single herb or method for eradicating viral infections. A virus has a protein coating. It has hooks. It can make enzymes that are able to penetrate the cell and dissolve its protective coating. Once inside the cell, it takes control of the host's metabolism. It will take command of the cell it invades, and direct the cell as it suits its own interest.

There are many different kinds of viruses. Mononucleosis is one of them; flu is another. In my opinion, viral infections are best met with natural home remedies, such as herbs, homeopathics, baths, and wet compresses.

How do you determine whether your sore throat is a strep infection or a viral infection?

- If your right shinbone is hotter than your left, it is likely that your sore throat comes from strep infection.
- Touch your cheekbone from nose to ears. If it is sore, it is more likely that your sore throat stems from strep infection.

Remedies for Infections

Viral infections—For influenza, put your loved one to bed. As with strep infection, give lots of fluids. Make a very good-tasting tea of two parts fennel, two parts thyme, one part lemon balm, and two parts rosehip.

Here is another good tea for all viral infections: Make a tea of two parts raspberry leaves, two parts nettle, one part roses, and one-half part echinacea.

Make a broth with white and red onions by boiling the onions in plenty of water. Cut medium-sized onions of each kind and simmer in one quart water until done. Remove from heat, strain, and give five tablespoons every hour, either straight or in water.

Colds, bad coughs, or pneumonia—Put right hand on patient's forehead, left hand on back of head. Hold ten minutes for a child, then drop hands to the chest and back for another ten minutes. Child will sleep away the illness. Also works for viral pneumonia in adults. The seat of pneumonia is in the head, not the lungs. For an adult, hold the above head posture for 20 minutes to half an hour. It is not necessary to hold the chest for adults. Do not hold tight or press, just lay on the hands. Hands will be wet at the end of the time period. Wash them. This is the poison leaving the body.

If a fever is involved, massage or put vinegar compresses on calves of the legs to draw the fever from the head to the legs.

Spanish thyme, good for the thymus gland, helps prevent colds. Take two cups of tea a day. Good in cooking. Add cream if children are reluctant to drink it. Can also add honey. Great beverage in winter months. For a cold or sinus congestion, avoid dairy products.

Coughs—Combine two parts thyme, one part sage, one part yarrow, and one part mullein.

Sinus infections—Take one teaspoon honey and sprinkle with freshly ground pepper. Eat it. This is also good for the sniffles.

Also, use yellow onion juice against any kind of cough. Take a yellow onion, make a good-sized hole on top. Fill with honey or raw sugar. The juice released is very helpful.

Use an herbal combination of lemon peel, chamomile, thyme, capsicum, coltsfoot, yerba santa, eucalyptus, wahoo bark, and mugwort.

Coxsackie

A physician in the town of Coxsackie, New York, found that many who suffer from pain in hip joints, hips, and lower back do not have arthritis, but have something caused by a virus. It is called Coxsackie, and this is a vicious disease. It takes a long time to manifest so that it becomes painful, but there is, as far as I know, only one remedy. The antidote comes from Dr. Ray (in England) and is called Coxsackie homeopathic. I am thoroughly amazed by how many people suffer from this virus. It is astounding that one small bottle of Coxsackie antidote can take away years and years of suffering.

Measles and Mumps

Measles and mumps are viral infections and should be treated with love and care, bed rest, warmth, light food, no ice water, no ice cream, warm oil on a painful cheek, and a darkened room. After having had measles, children are usually stronger.

Mononucleosis

A virus in the lymphatic system is widespread. You become tired, listless, sleepy, dull, and depressed. It can be with you for a long time, but it is easily taken care of with herbs. Try one quart of red raspberry tea daily.

Also, an herbal formula of raspberry leaves, basil, and lettuce will soon relieve this trouble. Be sure you take the herbs long enough. Mononucleosis goes into hiding only to break out when you don't expect it.

Arthritis

Dr. Douglas Baker from England tells us that most arthritis, osteoarthritis, and rheumatism have a hidden virus. In England, they found that a dog virus is responsible for these pains. In the United States, the herbal antidote is a combination of yucca, black walnut leaves, yellow dock, wormwood, and fenugreek seed. It is used to straighten out the damage.

This dog virus can be dormant for many, many years, only to break out whenever resistance is low.

Multiple Sclerosis

Medical researchers say the mysterious cause of multiple sclerosis (MS), the nerve-destroying disease that afflicts more than 250,000 Americans, could be the family dog. Dr. Stuart D. Cook, who is chief of the department of neurosciences at the College of Medicine and Dentistry in Newark, New Jersey, headed a team that investigated the possible link between dogs and MS.

In two separate studies, he surveyed 74 MS patients and matched them with people of the same age, sex, and socioeconomic level who did not have MS. He found that 65 of the 74 patients had pet dogs, while only 43 of the 74 MS-free people had them.

Dr. Cook reported his findings involving MS patients in the prestigious British medical journal *Lancet* and in the American Neurological Association's *Annals of Neurology*. Dr. Cook's research team also found that MS patients are more likely than other people to have dogs in both the five- and ten-year periods before the onset of the disease. Close exposure to pet dogs before the illness began was extremely high.

"These results suggest that exposure to housepets may sometimes be associated with subsequent MS," Dr. Cook concluded. Dr. Cook pointed out that distemper virus causes neurological damage in dogs, similar to the nerve-tissue destruction in human beings with MS. He said the findings also hold out hope for preventing MS.

Simian Virus 40

One of the biggest tragedies hit America in the late 1950s. It came like a shooting star, brilliant and beautiful. It raced from coast to coast, touching almost every home. Then it disappeared. But, unlike a shooting star, it left behind a trail of sorrow, despair, mental and physical illnesses, suicide, financial ruin for many families, and confusion. It was the Salk vaccine, the most extensive experiment on humans ever performed; and it became the biggest disaster ever known to mankind.

Thousands of little rhesus monkeys were shipped to America, delivered by the truckload to laboratories. Their little kidneys were pierced with long needles, and the deathly polio virus was injected. The little animals became deathly ill, their kidneys decomposing with pus and decay. At the height of their suffering, the rhesus monkeys were killed and the pus extracted. This was injected into fertile eggs and after a few days, the famous Salk vaccine was ready to be injected into our children's bloodstreams. Many vaccines are made that way; however, here entered the tragedy. The polio virus was dead, but no one knew or checked beyond that. With the vaccine, another little virus had slipped in, which is only known to be present in primates. This monkey virus has the scientific name of simian 40, in short sim 40 or SV40. Sim 40 is harmless to monkeys, but when entered into the bloodstream of our children, the disaster began.

Subsequent propaganda subdued the cries of the parents whose children were suddenly hit with, among other behavioral changes, the following symptoms:

- Fear
- Anguish
- Failing mental health
- Laziness
- Listlessness
- Hatred toward parents and teachers
- Lack of cleanliness
- Failing physical health
- Depression
- Low-grade temperature
- Meningitis

Many physicians quickly realized that something went wrong with the inoculations. To avoid more troubles for their patients, they injected sterile water until they knew what was going on, and the propaganda machine turned its focus to other things. It was Dr. Sabin to whom God gave the wisdom, stamina, and integrity to help us. Dr. Sabin also bought rhesus monkeys. One of his first helpers was bitten by one, and this man developed a strange fever. It looked just like a brain fever, but it was more than that and carried with it many of the symptoms that parents noticed in their inoculated children. Dr. Sabin found Sim 40 in his associate. Then he examined the Salk vaccine, and in each vial there was this monkey virus.

Sim 40 had never been in the human blood before, and all at once millions of Americans had it. Of course, many children were able to throw the virus off; but many of them, particularly the fine-nerved, sensitive children, were unable to cope with it. No one understood why these children behaved so strangely. They became loners; they were chilled, cold, and miserable. They became paranoid, fearful, and depressed, and they developed suicidal tendencies. In the streets they found company—boys and girls their age who understood what fear was. They all had the chill, they knew how terrible it was to be alone when the suicidal tendencies struck. They knew how the deep depression could hit and hurt.

> There can be few graver opportunities for manmade disaster than the mass immunization campaigns that are now routine in many countries. Should the vaccine preparations become contaminated with an undetected agent present in the host cells, such as a cancer-causing virus, a whole generation of vaccines could be put in jeopardy. This, of course, is no science fiction writer's horror story—it has already happened once; millions of people have been injected with a monkey virus known as SV40, which was found in 1961 to be contaminating polio and adenovirus vaccines. The virus causes cancer in hamsters; no one yet knows what it may do in man. (*Science*, 7 April 1972.)

The acute stage of this virus is over; however, it is not dead. The second episode is showing up. Many children, and even adults of all ages who may never have had the first inoculation of polio vaccine, now have Sim 40 in their systems. It hides in the spinal fluid and in the nervous system; they feel tension in the back of their necks and between the shoulder blades. According to medical textbooks, veterinarian textbooks, and the research done at Colorado University, Sim 40 is an RNA/DNA virus. That means it goes into the nervous system. It is the most feared of all types of viruses, because it can stay dormant for many years, just to strike whenever the system becomes low in energy.

One clairvoyant said, "I feel death in many people, right in their necks and between the shoulders."

Sim 40 may break up any day now and it is that which the Bible quotes: "When two stand in the fields, one will be taken."

I have searched and researched every avenue open to my simple mind and understanding. I have prayed for my own children and my beloved ones in the streets and mountains. Twenty-four years have passed and Sim 40 virus is still on the warpath. One of the factors leading to AIDS may have its roots in Sim 40.

A remedy:

Grind one-half pound basil, one-half pound kelp, and one pound milk sugar, and blend together. Take one teaspoon four times daily in water, juice, or yogurt for at least six weeks. I have noticed that some people have a light fever for a few days, but most people feel better right away for the first time in years. Also, a homeopathic product specific to Sim 40 is a miraculous help. Since this is a hidden virus, it may come and go for a while, but keep taking the formula. Watch your children regain their mental and physical stability. Watch yourself changing to better health.

I had a most unusual meeting with a physician from Switzerland. For a while she was the right hand of Dr. Albert Schweitzer, the "Saint of Lambaréné" (W. Africa). During the evening we talked about the hippie movement, and I told her the incredible story of Sim 40.

When I finished, the 80-year-old woman jumped to her feet, grabbed my shoulders, and said, "Say this once more. It cannot be, it cannot be."

I asked her why she was so excited and she answered, "Being with Dr. Schweitzer was the most incredible experience of my life. He helped everybody, he took everyone in, he treated animals, birds, and whatnot with utmost admiration for life itself; but when someone was bitten by an ape, he sent those people back into the jungles to die while tears ran down his cheeks. 'Ape virus, Sim 40,' he said, 'is a nerve virus. It settles in the RNA and DNA. It is also so dangerous to human blood that I cannot take the risk to have these people on my premises.'

"Sim 40 is still the pain in the neck."

Viroids

An entirely new field of infections is a newly discovered, tiny virus called *viroid*. Viroids can be 80 to 150 times smaller than a virus. They are ring shaped, and in contrast to a virus, they have no protein shell; they force themselves into a living cell. Viroids are able to give orders to the cell nucleus to reproduce viroids by the thousands.

It is entirely possible that viroid is latent in the cells, and it just breaks out when the environment is right. It is possible that the so-called slow viruses are indeed viroid. It is suggested by scientists that viroids may be in Alzheimer's disease, in nerve deterioration, in MS, and in other slow-progressing diseases. It is reported that viroid diseases are closely related to intron, and the disease appearance is similar.

Where do viroids come from? Are they genetic accidents, or normal components of a healthy cell that escape and pirate the cells of another species? No one has answers yet, but the speculations of viroid researchers led them to the frontiers of molecular biology—a rapidly evolving study that has lately revealed a surprisingly active and changeable life cycle for the nucleic acids RNA and DNA, which carry the genetic code. Biologists have found that these long-chain molecules often split apart and rearrange their internal parts. Theodor O. Diener, who coined the term *viroid*, speculates that the tiny pathogens are a kind of genetic fall-out from this process.

Can the human body harbor viroids? Yes, we can house these mystery agents. A viroid is so small that it cannot create or build an enzyme. Hans Gross of the Max Planks Institute in Munich was the first scientist to work out the genetic code of a spindle tube—a viroid. He surprised us with the most profound knowledge. A viroid (spindle tube) can contaminate a whole field of potatoes by hitching rides on tractor-drawn cultivators and then being brushed off onto other plants. Viroid diseases are also found in chrysanthemums. Called chloratic mottle, it also can destroy the citrus industry. This viroid is called an exocortis viroid and has done much damage.

Diener, an outstanding specialist on viroids, believes that they exist innocuously in some healthy plants and in tissue in tubes for a long time, only to become active for reasons unknown. Viroid researchers see no reason why some baffling animal and human diseases might not be caused by runaway fragments of RNA and DNA, which are viroids. Perhaps this is the case in Alzheimer's disease or other slow, progressive brain and spine disorders.

A viroid infection can be sudden, also. You feel fine one day, and the next day you feel as if you are two persons in one. Some people have double vision, most people feel very ill, and some experience backache. It can manifest in many ways. However, this invasion is seldom accompanied by a fever, so it is shrugged off, viewed as unimportant.

Viroids can become a new cancer in our lives. It is still not known what triggers activity. Could it be fallout? Could pollution, chemical saturation, or sodium fluoride be bringing new and crippling diseases? Scientists are studying the problem, and with the help of God, they will find the answer—a viroid antidote—in plants and humans.

Viroids can manifest in the following illnesses:

- Lymphoma
- Leukemia
- Norwalk virus
- Meningitis (both spinal and brain)

What to Do

To combat viroids, try the following remedies:

Viroid powder—Use a Viroid powder containing gelatin, rice polishings, whey, glutamic acid, and basil powder. Take one teaspoon twice daily in a glass of juice or water.

Aloe vera—This is the best. Take two leaves of an aloe vera plant, wash, and cut fine. Cover them with water, one cup aloe vera to three cups water. Bring to a boil and simmer for 15 minutes. Add one-half cup honey and simmer five more minutes. Take from the heat, cool, and strain. Take two tablespoons every hour for an adult, and one tablespoon every hour for a child. You may dilute it with water. The healing power seems to be in the green covering of the plant. It is excellent.

Viroid infections have a tendency to eat up your vitamin B_{12}; therefore, you become very tired during and after the infection.

Fungal Infections

A medical doctor recently stated that a problem of the future will be fungus. But this isn't a future problem; it's a problem now. It's a very common problem here in the United States, and many are plagued with it. Many lung problems are caused by fungus infections.

Candida Albicans

One of the most feared of all infections is the fungus infection. Over 2,000 years ago, Hippocrates described an oral and vaginal thrush that we know now as a fungus called Candida albicans. Normally, Candida albicans is confined to skin and mucous membranes but because of the general breakdown of our immune systems, Candida can also invade the bloodstream. Once in the bloodstream, it becomes a powerful poison that invades the nervous system.

Unrestrained Candida albicans occurs when this fungus takes off all at once. Candida albicans overgrowth means that this fungus has entered the bloodstream and no longer nests on membranes of the mouth or intestines. The following symptoms are caused by Candida albicans:

General:
- Fatigue
- Cold hands and feet
- Numbness and tingling
- Joint pains and stiffness
- Increased body hair

Gastrointestinal tract:
- Chronic heartburn
- Colitis
- Gas
- Gastritis
- Distention and bloating

Children with a yeast problem may exhibit the following symptoms (often following sugary meals or snacks):

- Hyperactivity
- Recurrent respiratory tract infections
- Recurrent ear infections
- Neurological and behavioral symptoms

The following symptoms may suggest a yeast problem in adults:

- Depression
- Prostatitis
- Hives
- Persistent vaginitis
- Digestive symptoms
- Psoriasis and other skin problems

- Extreme sensitivity to common chemicals such as perfumes or tobacco smoke
- Dysmenorrhea
- "Feeling bad all over" for no apparent reason
- Persistent jock itch
- Headaches
- Premenstrual syndrome
- Lack of coordination
- Impotence
- Athlete's foot and fungus growth on nails

When the poisonous effect of Candida albicans hits the central nervous system, we are in deep trouble. The fear of losing the mind is real, and many have suicidal tendencies and so on.

The following are just a few of the signs that the fungus Candida albicans is in its final stage:

- Headaches
- Lethargy
- Memory loss
- Depression
- Hyperirritability
- Inability to concentrate

This is a serious problem. Fifty percent of all people in mental institutions suffer acutely from this fungus infection. Out of 169 adults studied, 163 had Candida albicans overgrowth. Candida albicans occurs in everyone, but a healthy body keeps it in its natural limits, and it causes no harm.

Bob, a teenager, had a serious acne problem. The only thing that helped him was tetracycline. He had taken it for two years with only minor pauses in between. The acne subsided, but left huge scars on his face. I met him when he was 20—he was depressed and shy; leaned toward drinking; had cold hands and feet; complained of stomach trouble, bleeding ulcers, and bleeding bowels; and at times, he was tremendously restless.

For a minor incident in a bar he was sent to a penitentiary. Because of his restlessness and depression, he was placed in a crawlspace where he could not stand up or walk but could just lie or sit on the floor. After three weeks in that dungeon, he had to be put in the hospital and chained to his bed. Released, he never found his way back. He was a plumber (and a good one), but he did it without joy or enthusiasm. The money he made he used for the only relief of his depression—dope. He died of an overdose, eight hours before his little son was born. Cause of death: Candida albicans, the fungus activated by tetracycline in his teens.

What to Do

Use the following diet and lifestyle suggestions to combat Candida albicans:

- Eat a low-carbohydrate diet. Buy a carbohydrate guide so you can keep track of your intake.

- Avoid antibiotics and steroids unless absolutely necessary.

- Do not use birth control pills if you fear this problem. The pills upset hormones, thus interfering with the body's ability to fight Candida.

- Take up to three tablets or capsules of acidophilus and/or bifidis each meal.

- Use garlic. If you cannot eat the whole garlic, take an odorless garlic supplement.

- At least 30,000 IU of vitamin A should be used for the first two weeks of this program. Thereafter, cut the dosage down to 24,000 IU per day. (Use the emulsified form of vitamin A for the high dosage segment. It will not accumulate in your liver.)

- B$_{15}$ seems to be effective.

- Approximately two weeks into the program, add two tablets per meal of raw thymus, a glandular tissue.

- Use quaw bark tincture to uplift the immune system.

- Take three to six zinc tablets at a strength of 15 mg daily.

- Try an herbal combination of white pine bark, mugwort, myrrh, chamomile, catnip, and mullein. Take with meals.

- A combination of condurango bark, yellow dock, and red clover is another herbal antidote to Candida albicans. This should be taken with an herbal combination of tansy, clay, milkweed, cramp bark, goldenseal leaves, and blessed thistle.

- Drink five ounces of marjoram tea twice a day.

- Exercise at least 20 minutes a day.
- Moderate sunlight is beneficial in killing candida overgrowth.
- Reduce the intake of refined carbohydrates and alcohol.
- Avoid all yeast products.
- Avoid brewer's yeast, raw mushrooms, chocolate, and other sweets.

Fungus in Lungs

Cases of fungus in the lungs are more and more frequent. Fungus is like a mushroom. When you cut a batch of mushrooms, two days later a new batch is growing a few yards away. The feelers, the spores, just grow a new batch. The same holds true with mushrooms in your system. We call this metastasis. What can you do to change your chemistry so that fungus will be discouraged to grow? Change your diet.

Cancer

"Cancer is a disease of the RNA/DNA structure of the cell," the medical books tell us. "Cancer is not a single disease but a group of many diseases with a common characteristic; uncontrolled, invasive growth at the expense of normal body system, but the basic cause of cancer is unknown," they conclude.

Not so. We know that cancer is a fungus disease, and in rare cases it is a spindle cell viroid. Since cancer, in most cases, is a fungus disease, we have to determine which foods and herbs are antifungal in nature.

Never toss away the helping hand of a surgeon who is able to remove a cancerous growth, but try not to let it reach this point. If it does, remove the growth, but do something afterwards. Change your lifestyle by cleaning the fungi from your body. Do something against metastasis: Make your diet consist of 50 percent raw food, 50 percent cooked food, and NO protein after 2 P.M.

What to Do

Follow these guidelines to help in the fight against cancer:

- No more fried, greasy foods
- No more TV dinners
- No more aluminum pots, pans, or foil
- No more soft drinks or beer from aluminum cans
- No more protein after 2 P.M.
- No more pastry and sugar products
- Food has to be 50 percent raw and 50 percent cooked

To change body chemistry fast, drink one gallon of hyssop tea sweetened with honey or maple sugar for a day. No other foods. If at all possible, do it two days in a row.

The following foods are antifungal:

- Asparagus: Take two tablespoons cooked asparagus (can be canned) two to three times daily.
- Alfalfa sprouts are very good to stop cancerous growth.
- Almonds contain B_{17}.
- Macadamia nuts are rich in B_{17}.
- Onion: Parboil and use in salads and foods.
- Seeds: Flaxseed, chia seed, sesame seed, and clover seed.
- Grains: Oat groats, barley, buckwheat groats, millet, and rye.
- Beans: Lentils, mung beans, and chick peas.

The following herbs are antifungal:

- Combine red clover blossoms, cascara sagrada bark, chaparral, sarsaparilla, licorice root, prickly ash bark, pokeroot, burdock root, peach bark, buckthorn bark, Oregon grape root, Norwegian kelp, and stillingia.
- An herbal combination of alfalfa seed, blessed thistle, and golden-seal root is a powerful herb food combination often used with and after antibiotics. It is a fungus infection transmuter. Combine

ELECTROMAGNETIC FOOD COMBINATIONS
This diet is important to fight cancer.

1
- All seafood
- Whole eggs
- Lamb
- Beef
- Potatoes, white
- Potatoes, sweet
- Eggs
- Veal
- Oyster
- All fish
- Olive oil
- Rutabagas
- Tomatoes, fresh
- Tomatoes, cooked
- Green pepper
- Rice
- Oils

2
- Spinach
- Avocado
- Watercress
- Okra
- Beets
- Radishes
- Parsnips
- Salsify
- Lettuce
- Sauerkraut
- Kohlrabi
- Beet tops
- Dandelion
- Brussels sprouts
- Peppermint
- Broccoli
- Green peas
- Cauliflower
- Carrots
- Green corn
- Onions
- Watercress
- Green beans
- Cabbage
- Escarole
- Asparagus
- Pumpkin
- Cucumbers
- Chard

3
- Sweet milk, raw
- Yogurt
- Cream
- Filberts
- Tea, lemon
- Gelatin
- Bread, whole grain
- Steel cut oats
- Cereals
- Cornmeal
- Maple syrup
- Almonds
- Wheat germ
- Goat's milk, raw
- Buttermilk
- Cheese, natural
- Butter
- Cottage cheese
- Millet
- Rice
- Bread

4
- Cherries
- Apricots
- Peaches
- Pineapple
- Grapes
- Plums
- All berries
- Bananas
- Melons
- Molasses
- Brown sugar
- Preserves, honey
- Raisins
- Dates
- Figs
- Pomegranates
- Currants
- Rice, brown

5a
- Lentils
- Beans, dried
- Mushrooms
- Peas, dried
- Eggplant
- Peanuts

5b
- Grapefruit
- Lemons
- Limes
- Watermelon

5c
- Cooked or canned
- Tomatoes
- Spaghetti
- Rice
- Corn
- Millet

Combine:
- Combine 1 and 2
- Combine 3 and 4
- Combine 5a with 2
- + Corn, Rice, Millet, Greens above ground
- Combine 5c with 2
- Apples and rice are universal

it with an herbal combination of yellow dock, cramp bark, yarrow, milkweed, plantain, organic tobacco, and tansy; this acts as a blood cleanser.

- To reduce the "feelers" is the next job. (This recipe is used in Europe.) Take one and a half cups milk, add two tablespoons dried calendula petals. Bring to a boil and simmer for ten minutes. Strain it. The herb milk is a day's supply.

- For fungus on toenails or fingernails, try this method. Take kerosene and add camphor (available in drugstores as a white block.) Chop camphor block into kerosene until saturated, then paint nails with this solution twice daily. After a week, nails improve.

I want to introduce to you the outstanding work of Dr. H. Budwig, from Germany. This doctor offers practical help in her book, *Is Cancer a Fat Problem?* She said, "Cancer patients have to eat, but starve the tumors." Her method is to take raw cottage cheese called "quark" and add cold-pressed oils to it. With this, the starved cells are supplied with an oxygen-rich product.

Her findings coincide with those of Dr. Szent-Györkis's research, even though they never met. Both physicians say that certain proteins can carry electrons that are vital for the health of starving cells. With raw oil, Dr. Budwig adds another important factor—vitamin F—which also becomes an oxygen carrier to the starving cells.

Self-Examination Taught in England and Denmark

Sterilize a pin, then prick a fingertip. When the blood appears pearl-like, you are healthy. When it smears, you need to change your diet and lifestyle. When the drop runs and more than several drops come out from one prick in a thin stream, have an examination by a doctor, change your diet, get well quickly, and thank God for this knowledge.

Self-Examination Taught in America

Put part of your morning urine in a smooth plastic cup. Cover it with one thin layer of tissue paper and set in a dark place, such as under the sink or cupboard. At bedtime set the cup in your refrigerator on the lowest shelf, way back so that no one else touches it. Next morning, pour urine out. If you have a fungus in your system there will be a fatty, waxy rim where urine and air meet. This is an early examination that you can do for yourself.

Leukemia

Leukemia does not have the characteristics of a fungus disease. Professor Brauchle in Dresden taught and demonstrated the following: "I want to illustrate to you the cause of leukemia. Here is my little dog. Take a blood sample and examine it. Then treat the dog badly for one week. Scold him, turn him away, but give him food as before."

After one week the dog had leukemia. The next week we were to be kind to him and love him. No extra food was permitted. When his blood was tested, no leukemia was found. Brauchle taught us this lesson, remarking that "it is the same with animals as it is with humans." Some children do not get enough love, others reject love, and both are heading for leukemia.

What to Do

Under Brauchle's guidance, we had to stroke the children from head to toe lightly, ever so lightly, hardly touching the body. I was amazed to learn that this is not done all over the world. We also prepared the following egg fruit drink:

1 pt. freshly squeezed orange juice
1 pt. freshly squeezed grapefruit juice
1 pt. water with the juice of 3 limes
1 pt. water with the juice of 2 lemons
1 pt. frozen pineapple juice, diluted

1 pt. papaya juice, diluted
1 pt. grape juice
12 whole eggs
6 egg yolks
Frozen raspberries or strawberries to add a delicious flavor

Beat eggs and mix into fruit mixture. This is one day's supply. For a child, give a third to a half of the above amount. Beating of the eggs and egg yolks seems to be very important. Eggs prepared this way will remove avidin from the stomach.

What Is B_{17}?

B_{17} is not a newcomer. It has been used for a long time. Researchers found B_{17} in over 1,000 plants. It is present in the most concentrated form in bitter almonds and apricot kernels, but millet and all seeds show B_{17} in appreciable amounts.

The Chinese used bitter almond tea for tumors as far back as 3,500 years ago. It has been used in the Eastern world for centuries as an extract, a tea, and an infusion. In Turkey, apricot kernels are combined with figs and given as a special treat for cancer patients.

The Greeks and Romans used bitter almond water medicinally and called it *Amygdala amara*. As early as 1845, Fedor Inosemozov, the Russian physician, combined bitter and sweet almonds for two kinds of "fungus-like tumors."

In 1830, the chemists Robiquot and Boutyron isolated B_{17}, called amygdalin, in its pure form. Only seven years later, in 1837, the scientists Liebig and Woehler discovered that amygdalin is split by an enzyme complex into one molecule of hydrogen cyanide, one molecule of benzaldehyde, and two molecules of sugar.

Commercially, B_{17} is called laetrile, and a tremendous cloud hangs over this word. Laetrile has two aspects when specially fabricated. The laetrile from Mexico has a positive male vibration, and the laetrile from Germany has a female vibration.

I suggest that you make your own B_{17}, which is cheap and most effective, and it also has both male and female aspects; therefore, the body can and will pick up the vibration it needs.

Recipe for B$_{17}$:
    4 apricot kernels
    2 pieces dried apricot
    5 tablets *Calcarea carbonica* 6x homeopathic or limewater

Chew this. Take the formula twice daily. It tastes wonderful!

Color Healing—Let There Be Light...

The pineal gland converts light energy into an electrochemical impulse that feeds directly into the hypothalamus. The hypothalamus is filled with chromophilic (light-sensitive) cells that convert the electromagnetic signal of light into a neurochemical impulse. This is then carried directly to the pituitary gland. The pineal gland acts as a general synchronizing, stabilizing, and moderating organ on behalf of several physiological processes.

In the New Age, healing will be done through music and color. Music and color have been used throughout history by the Egyptians, Hebrews, and Greeks. Color healing provides a tremendous uplift to the immune and lymphatic systems, and acts as an antidote to inflammations and infections. Color healing is gentle and very effective. It becomes an even greater tool if used in conjunction with music—but not music with loud voices and many instruments.

ATTRIBUTES OF SPECTRO-CHROMO COLORS

Red   Stimulates the nervous system, which energizes sight, smell, taste, hearing, and touch. Stimulates and energizes the liver and builds hemoglobin. Makes you feel warm and energetic, and expels poisons from the system through the skin.

Orange   Stimulates the lungs—a lung builder. Stimulates the thyroid and relieves cramps and muscular spasms. Helps stomach glands to work properly and relieves flatulence. Best of all, corrects bone softness and rickets and helps calcium to be absorbed properly.

Yellow   Stimulates the motor nervous system, which energizes the muscles. Helps the lymphatic system, which becomes sluggish due to the scanners in the grocery stores. Stimulates bile production and influences pancreatic enzyme output. Therefore, it increases bowel movements. Increases peristaltic movements and even makes worms and parasites so uncomfortable that they leave. Is used in melancholia because it functions as an equilibrator by balancing portal circulations.

Lemon   Works by being a cerebral stimulant. Therefore, it favorably changes the process of nutrition (assimilation) and can repair old, persistent disorders. It's a bone builder because it brings phosphorus into action. It's a thymus stimulant and can become a good expectorant when mucous congests lungs and bronchia.

Green   A pituitary stimulant. It influences muscle and tissue building. May dissolve blood clots and should always be tried when clots are forming. Destroys bacteria, viruses, and viroids. Acts as a germicide and disinfectant. Prevents decay and is a fine cleanser.

Turquoise   See **Blue.**

Blue   A pineal stimulant; therefore, it builds vitality. Reduces fever (febrifuge). Removes inflammation. Relieves itching and is very soothing to the nervous system. Relieves burns and is cooling and refreshing.

Indigo   A parathyroid stimulant; therefore, it makes calcium available to the nervous system and acts as a tranquilizer. Checks the flow of blood because more calcium is freed to act on blood corpuscles and platelets. It's a pain reliever. Eases suffering caused by grief, excitement, and uncertainty. Acts as a sedative.

Violet   A spleen stimulant. Builds white blood cells to defend against infections. Decreases overstimulated muscular activity (hyperactivity) and also calms down overactive heart muscle. It's a lymph gland depressant, which comes in handy in mononucleosis or other lymph diseases.

Purple   Increases the function of the veins. Lowers blood pressure by dilating the blood vessels, reducing heart rate, and helping the kidneys. Reduces fever and makes you less sensitive to pain. Induces relaxation and gives you deep sleep.

Magenta   It's an aura builder. It stabilizes emotions. Stimulates heart, kidney, and adrenal gland. Increases circulation and makes you feel happy.

Scarlet   Contracts the blood vessels; therefore, it increases blood pressure. It's helpful when delivering a baby, because it tends to expel the infant easily. Increases kidney functions.

Color and Sound

When color is used just as a color, it is to the body as a day without a breeze. The color cannot penetrate to stimulate the pituitary or the kidney because there is no sound to guide the color deeper into the respective organ.

When you use sound, it has to be the sound of one melody performed by one instrument, such as one voice or one viola or one cello or one violin. If an orchestra plays during color healing, the aura will close and the well-intended music will not heal and will not bring the color to work.

This is what you do: Buy solo pieces or sing yourself. Make your own recording in the following way:

Color	Sound (music piece) in	Color	Sound
Red	G	Orange	A
Yellow	A#	Lemon	B
Green	C	Turquoise	C#
Blue	D	Indigo	D#
Violet	E	Purple	A#
Magenta	G and E	Scarlet	G

Color healing should be accompanied by the sound of one voice or the tone of one violin or one cello. No wonder the lullabies we sang to our children were so soothing, so effective. One sound brings colors into the aura. Sound and color will be the future healing therapy.

❧ CHAPTER SEVEN ❧

Miasm and Residue As a Cause of Ill Health

"The environment you fashion out of your thoughts…your beliefs…your ideals…your philosophy…is the only climate you will ever live in."
— Alfred Armond Montepert

"The only source of knowledge is experience."
— Albert Einstein

Miasms are carried-over diseases that have their genetic origin in long-past forefathers. A miasm can be traced to four and five generations before you. The disease pattern is not the same as the original disease, and it tends to be very hard to treat with conventional or unconventional methods. I know for sure of three distinct miasms:

- Tuberculosis (TB)
- Syphilis
- Gonorrhea

These days, people speak of cancer miasms and others. Remember, a miasm has its origin long ago, but it expresses in this lifetime in a completely different form.

TB miasms express themselves in the following ways:

- Scoliosis
- Hammertoe
- Bunions
- Enlarged, painful finger joints that we call arthritis
- Weak lungs, but which hardly ever manifest tuberculosis

Remedies for Miasms

TB residue responds to a homeopathic specific to TB residue, rubbed into painful areas and taken by mouth.

Lupus also seems to have its origin way back, and is helped by taking a TB residue-specific homeopathic and *Thuja occidentalis* homeopathic. It takes three years to interrupt this miasm.

Syphilis miasm goes still farther back. As all miasms, it skips a generation or two to appear in skin lesions, general weakness, psoriasis, and dementia. *Syphonium* homeopathic is the answer.

Gonorrhea miasm is the least serious one, and good nutrition is the factor indicated here.

Inoculations That Leave Undesirable Residues

Tetanus:	Constrictive nature, particularly in babies (crybabies)
Measles:	Nerves in spine and trouble in spinal fluid; MS
Mumps:	Female cysts and most often a cause of prostrate trouble in later life

Mumps and measles residues can be carried over from childhood when these diseases are not cared for in a proper manner (warmth, rest, and love). The virus can hide and strike mercilessly when men and women are in the prime of life.

In this category go the hidden, subtle poisons that humankind has to deal with, such as the following:

Black widow:	Nerve poison
Brown spider:	Nerve poison
Dog bite:	Convulsions, even years and years later
Rattler:	Of constrictive nature, often in throat, producing constant cough or heart pain (poison can be in milk, cheese, or meat from an animal bitten by a rattlesnake)

Your Tool: The Pendulum

I first learned about the pendulum through Linda Clark, a famous author on nutrition. In her book *Get Well Naturally*, she describes how her friends used the pendulum, and that is where it all started. I took my wedding ring and hung it on a thread, dangling it over my hands, my knees, and my food. Slowly, the ring started gyrating. I steadied myself in every possible way, but the ring was moving.

For one year I worked on this phenomenon, not showing it to anyone but my closest friends. I ordered books from England, France, and America. I found writings in the Bible about it. I talked to prominent women, to doctors, to psychologists, but no one could give me the answers I was searching for. Why does a pendulum work? What energies are involved? There are many more questions.

About Vibrations

We live in three worlds of vibrations. The first manifestation of vibration is physical and expresses in:

- feeling
- audible sound
- subsonic sound
- supersonic sound

These manifestations are transmitted through gas, liquids, and solids. The speed of transmission through these media is 1,100 feet per second (fps) in air. Physicists and scientists have instruments to measure the physical existence of these vibrations.

The second manifestation of vibration is electromagnetic in nature. It's expressed in the following:

- Low frequency electrical
- Radar high frequency
- Ultraviolet rays
- Radio broadcast
- Infrared
- Cosmic rays

These vibrations are transmitted through the ether at a speed of approximately 185,000 miles per second.

In 1975, scientists declared that the human body has an electromagnetic system with circuits and outlets. Vibrations use this electromagnetic system. Even though it is possible for the scientists to measure vibrations outside the body, it is not possible as yet to measure these frequencies in the human body with conventional methods and instruments.

The human body has organs that transform the electromagnetic waves so that the impact is buffered. These organs are the holy chakras. There are nine chakras in Westerners, eight in Native Americans, and seven in Easterners.

The third manifestation of vibration is astral-etheric in nature. It is called Higher Dimensional Energies (HD), and is expressed in the following:

- Aura emanations
- Meditation
- Emotions
- ESP (extrasensory perception)
- Eloptic emanations
- Prayers
- Thoughts

The medium through which these vibrations are transmitted is Akashic or Nieonic. The speed of transmission through this medium is instantaneous.

Physicists and chemists, including biochemists, do not have the proper instruments to measure etheric vibrations. Even the De La Warr's Radionic Instruments need an operator with well-developed ESP.

Intuition comes from a higher realm. Intuition is the language of the soul. If you could find an instrument with which you could speak to your soul directly, would that not be a fantastic invention? Such an instrument exists. It is the pendulum. (Your soul is always connected to a higher intelligence—God.) Question your soul with your pendulum, and you will receive the answer through your pendulum.

Some scientists will admit that there are aura emanations. Some will admit that there is power in mantras and prayers. However, scientists do not have an instrument that will measure the output of an earnest prayer. There is no gadget that can measure a prayer in numbers or weight or angstroms. Therefore, scientists may deny the existence of these powers. They will deny the reading of an aura meter or a psychometric reading, and will ridicule the use of a dowsing rod.

Many people think that what scientists cannot measure does not exist. That is not so. The foundation on which science stands is the rational, materialistic realm. The prayer of a soul and the purity of a heart are realms of a higher nature, beyond the rational, materialistic view.

In many areas of the United States, radiesthesia is still a public no-no. This is hard to believe since radiesthesia is widely and publicly used in France, England, Germany, and Russia. In particular, France, because of pioneer Abbe Mermet, is way ahead in psychometric knowledge. And yet, it was in America that the greatest breakthrough into the realization of these astral-etheric vibrations was made. Scientists found that the nerves are transmitters of the previously mentioned vibrations. In 1975, it was recognized that the electromagnetic web below the skin could transmit energies.

In 1908, researchers at Harvard University came up with astounding news. They found that certain energies enter our bodies through the pores of the skin, go through endless nadis or channels, and gather in 33 centers. I want to make sure that we understand that these higher energies are not electromagnetic in nature—they are not using the chakras as transformers. They are finer in nature. These energies are true healers.

Through these nadis and centers the intuition flows. As previously indicated, the intuition is the language of the soul, and the pendulum, the rod, and radiesthesia are the instruments with which you can measure, verify, and interpret the language of your soul and come in contact with the all-knower.

At Harvard, the research was dropped because they had no practical use for it.

ᵉ CHAPTER EIGHT ᵉ

Electromagnetism

Healing with magnetism is the oldest form of healing known to mankind. The Kabbalah teaches it, the old Hindu healing system taught it, and it was taught in the mystery schools of the Orient and Occident. We are very much inclined to call it suggestive healing, but there is more to it than suggestion. Goethe said: "Magnetism is an all-present, all-reaching power. Every human being has it. Only according to the human individuality it differs in strength. Its action works on everything and magnetism is everywhere."

Every mother has the urge to place her hand over her youngster's feverish forehead, aching back, or sore thumb. We do not have to doubt any longer that a power leaves our hands. Kirlian photography proves that.

The electromagnetic force field is not the only energy that can be employed and used for healing. There is prana energy, which penetrates each cell of our body and flows from East to West. There is also the so-called sun-moon energy that is expressed in certain people, and this is a gift of the Divine to which I know only one fitting key. It is to work on the development of your light within. When path and goal are one, this power will develop.

We have long been aware that our bodies have both a positive and a negative side. Much has been written on this. We have polarity and magnetic healing. Both use the negative and the positive, but neither opens the flow of electromagnetic power to the organs. The head is the control tower, and the neck is the magnetic keyboard for the entire body.

Magnetism is a natural energy. Earth itself is a giant magnet with positive and negative poles. Forces released by the magnetic North Pole encircle Earth, and as we know, the energies affect all living things. We are bathed in this electromagnetic force field, and no life would exist without it. Scientists tell us that magnetism is generated in the atoms. That means that we, too, are magnets.

We are magnetic generators. We live on top of a magnet in the influence of magnetic energies of other planets and worlds, and we still know very little about this subject. I believe it was Einstein who said, "The knowledge about that which we know is only a fraction from that which we do not know." In fact, when it comes to the healing arts and magnetism, the subject is called a *dark force*, *witchcraft*, or a *special gift*, and its results are called *unbelievable* or *unreal*. It is condemned and ridiculed, but it has remained with us since mankind began. It was not previously known why the laying on of hands helped, but now, because of the work of many scientists, we do know. This book is a guide for everyone who is willing to help his fellow man.

The entire body is a field of flowing electromagnetic energy. Wherever this flow stops, for one reason or another, we have a short circuit, and the pattern of life and health is impaired.

The laying on of hands in the right manner may aid in bringing back the energy to full flow, and may repair the short circuit. To understand how this works, we have to know the exact manner and flow of the human biomagnetic energies.

Magneto Therapy: The Laying On of Hands

The laying on of hands is as old as humankind itself. Why, then, did it come to be so discredited when the Kabbalah teaches it in detail and the Indians used it in their Vedic system of healing? The primitives used it, and Jesus Christ used it. Furthermore, Jesus said, "This and more thou shall do in my name."

In the Middle Ages, the laying on of hands was mainly practiced by kings and rulers. It was a royal art. Edward III, for example, was considered a supersaint. He reportedly healed 136 people in one afternoon session. Frederick Barbarossa was a healing king. Charlemagne was called a saint because of the many healings that took place under his hands.

The House of the Habsburgs had many fine healing kings. Maximilian, who died in the year 1519, had such outstanding healing qualities that many celebrities of other countries came to pay him a visit in order to be healed.

The House of Burgundy (France) also had outstanding healing kings. They were called Sons of God's Grace. One of the best known healers was

Charles X. He reportedly healed 128 people in one afternoon with the famous phrase, "The King touches you, and God heals you." Philip I was very successful in healing scrofula, which is, we know now, a deficiency disease.

Basically, the kings touched the foreheads of their subjects and made the sign of the cross. Many times they used holy water that they made themselves. The ritual for making holy water was a secret, and it was handed down from father to son, from ruler to ruler, and from generation to generation. Finally, holy water was partially adopted by the churches.

At that time there was no conflict between the ruling kings and the medics. Every royal family employed medics. Healing by a king was not a cure-all. It was considered an act of God, performed through the hands of the king.

How Does It Work?

The front right side of the body is positive; the left side is negative. The magnetic poles in the human body are just below the navel. There it is neutral. Over the sex organs, there is a strong positive biomagnetic field.

Previously we thought that the spine was the neutral point, the magnetic pole, but after studying the knowledge of the Kabbalah, I found that the ancients knew differently, and by measuring these points I found it to be true. This knowledge is of great significance, and the laying on of hands becomes a science of great importance.

The backside of the body is more complicated. The back of the head has a strong positive biomagnetic field. Also, the base of the spine is strongly positive. In between these two positive poles, the spine is negatively charged. The right kidney is positive. The left kidney is negative. The right shoulder plate is positive. The left shoulder plate is negative. The right hip is positive. The left hip is negative.

In order to achieve results, we have to turn our full attention to our work. With every stroke, with every movement, we should realize the healing power of the Divine.

We need to realize that we are able to increase results by increasing the power of our minds, to which there is no limitation. A concentrated thought pattern releases energies that become vital and necessary for magneto therapy. There is no need to undress anyone. We need to release the anxiety and not increase it by embarrassment.

In acute cases and in nervous disorders, we can reduce the electromagnetic activity with the soothing power of the left hand. In all healing crises that may occur, we again work with the left hand and give support to the magnetic pole with the right hand.

The duration of the treatment is between five and ten minutes. In acute cases, it should be done every day. In other cases, it only needs to be done once a week.

Magneto therapy is not new, but the understanding of the electromagnetic poles and the proper placement of the hands are new. New also is the understanding of positive and negative ions. New are discoveries of electromagnetic functioning of the very cells of the different parts of the body—the blood as an electromagnetic stream of power and the nervous system as the tract for speedy delivery of electromagnetic impulses. All this knowledge is new and exciting.

Magneto therapy is not meant to replace and will not take away the need for a physician, a surgeon, or a hospital. It is not meant to replace and will not eliminate the need for a proper diet or medicine. It is not a replacement for vitamins or minerals. But it will increase the ability to live in a poisoned world more efficiently. It will bring into balance the delicate electromagnetic system without which we cannot exist.

There are times when it is needed as an emergency, and always and in all cases, the treatments only complement the work of a physician.

Magneto therapy can never injure or hurt, but only strengthen the healing process that takes place in every organism. Remember, no one heals but God and nature. Every healing attempt is only a little help to the healing process taking place through the power of the Divine.

Magneto therapy always influences the whole body. Children are often restless, nervous, lacking in energy, moody, or fearful. The cause may be a malfunctioning organ, lack of a certain nutrient, or intoxication by heavy metals. A physician will find the cause. An electromagnetic treatment in all cases will harmonize the nervous system and the organs. God is law and order, and when we follow these laws of guiding, directing, and organizing the unordered, distorted, sick electromagnetic body into the order of the universe, health will result.

There are three fundamental stroke patterns, three distinct movements to use in the laying on of hands:

- Parallel or straight stroke
- Spiral
- Circle or loop

The parallel or straight stroke movement mainly influences the digestive tract. The spiral movement influences mostly the nervous system. The circle movement is not closed, but an open loop. Do this for the heart, lungs, and congested areas.

No part of the body is active unless magnetic energy flows to it. This flow of magnetic energy is the basic principle of magnetic healing.

A schooled magneto therapist is capable of relieving conditions of pain and discomfort with only one or two treatments. The hands must be dry. No magnetic flow can take place with wet hands. Rub your hands together until they are hot. Then place the fingertips of your right hand in the palm of your left hand. Stand on tiptoe and will the electromagnetic powers to go through you and over you. This takes only 45 to 60 seconds. Then your body is tuned in to the magnetic flow.

Always keep your mind positive. Imagine perfect health and realize that you become a tool for the powers of the universe and a servant to the Lord. A great help was given to me by Dr. Doreal. He said to imagine the flow of magnetism increasing and flowing very rapidly. I learned to increase the flow of electromagnetism by imagination. I visualize a little brook, a small amount of water trickles down, and as I hold my hands, I imagine the increase of water in the brook until it is a complete and mighty flow unobstructed by stones or branches. Washing away obstacles of all kinds is the idea.

The Parallel or Straight Stroke

To work with the biomagnetic forces, please do not undress your patient. Let him take off his shoes and make his feet feel comfortable. A well-padded massage table is best. A couch or a mat on the floor will do.

Stand on the right side of your friend and tell him to close his eyes and to concentrate on the light within, the healing power of Christ within, or the electromagnetic power of the universe. Tell him that he is a child of the universe, subject to the universal laws and powers.

Remember, your right hand is positive so it has to stroke the left side of your friend's body. The left hand is negative, so it will stroke the right side. The strokes have to be very light in nature, slow in character, with the thumbs two inches apart. You start from the head down, but leave the crown of the head untouched. Go particularly slowly over trouble areas such as the liver and intestines. Concentrate intensely on your work, and realize and feel the balance you are bringing back.

When you arrive at the hips, you swing out, shake your hands, and in a wide movement, draw your hands back to the head. (Shaking of hands and the wide semicircle is needed to break the magnetic current.) Never let your hands glide back over the body to the head. You would undo with a single stroke all the strokes previously done.

Keep this up for three to four minutes. This procedure is fundamental in all magneto therapy movements. They should always be the first strokes you do. They normalize and harmonize the digestive tract and balance all electromagnetic functions in general.

If you want to stimulate the body, use the right hand only. The right hand adds fire to the magnetic system.

Place your left hand on top of your friend's head. Stroke with the right hand from head to toe. For a tall person, you have to let him flex his knees so you can reach the toes without taking your hand off the head. The stroke has to sweep off the toes. Shake your hand, and using a wide semicircle, bring it back up to the head.

The Spiral Stroke

With the spiral movement, we influence the entire nervous system. Have your friend lie comfortably on a well-padded massage table. Again, do not remove clothes. Only the shoes and heavy coats are removed. You are not giving a Swedish massage. You are dealing with higher powers, and we know they penetrate the material covering of your spirit's vehicle, your body.

For a stimulating effect, needed for instance when the person is in a depressed state or feeling low vitality in general, place your left hand over the head, and with your right hand perform clockwise spiral motions over the body from head to toe. The spiral has to have the circumference of the width of the body.

Having arrived at the toes, shake your hand, and with a wide swinging motion, come back to the head and perform this movement for three to five minutes.

A calming effect will be achieved by placing the right hand over the toes (point fingers in the direction of the toes), while the left hand performs counterclockwise spirals from the head over the toes. Shake your hands, and in a wide semicircle, come back to the top of the head.

The Circle Stroke

The circle movement is a little open loop. It is a small movement not larger than a silver dollar.

The counterclockwise circle is performed with your left hand, and it is soothing and calming. The clockwise circle is performed with your right hand, and it is stimulating. The duration of the circular movement should be one to two minutes, never longer. This technique is used after you use the first and/or second technique—the straight stroke and/or the spiral stroke.

This movement is mainly used for bringing heart, lung, liver, and circulation into balance and harmony. It is also used to close energy leaks and to open congestion of various kinds.

Decongestion and Stimulation with Magneto Therapy

Magneto therapy can also stimulate and decongest the body. Use the following methods for the specified problem areas.

Stimulation of Heart

To stimulate the heart, place your left hand on top of your friend's head. With the right hand, perform 70 small, open, clockwise loops per minute. You can also do this to yourself. Start at the left side of your head and come down doing a loop over the neck and over the entire sternum around the heart. After the 70th stroke, shake your hand, go back to the starting point, and repeat the process.

These little open circles or loops must be featherweight in touch, and the sicker the person, the lighter the stroke must be. In severe cases, you hardly touch the body and perform another "loop treatment." Use a less firm stroke two hours later.

When you want to calm the heartbeat, place your right hand on your friend's knees (drawn up) and perform 70 loops per minute with your left hand, counterclockwise in the previously described manner.

Stimulation of Breathing

To stimulate the lungs and breathing, follow this procedure. Again, place your left hand on top of your own or your friend's head. With your right hand, start at the right side in clockwise movements of 18 circles per minute; come down the side of the neck, over the right shoulder, cover the entire chest, then return to the starting point. Repeat once more.

Soothing-Calming

For a calming effect, place your right hand on the toes of your friend. Point the fingers in the direction of the toes. The left hand makes the strokes from the head over the toes. Shake your hands and in a wide semi-circle, then come back to the top of the head.

Another way is to place your right hand on the drawn-up knees of your friend and with the left hand perform the circle movement in a counter-clockwise loop.

Decongest Your Gallbladder

The small circle method is used to open up congested areas. An example is a blocked-up gallbladder. Do this 18 times clockwise with the right hand. For an infected gallbladder, do this 18 times counterclockwise with the left hand.

Constipation

With the right hand, stroke clockwise 70 times per minute. Follow the large intestine, with the left hand on top of the head.

Stimulation of Circulation

To stimulate circulation, place your left hand on top of the stomach, finger pointing down. With your right hand stroke the left leg with parallel strokes from the groin, down the left leg, and over the foot. Interrupt the magnetic lock by shaking hand and in a wide semicircle start at the groin down. Alternate the hands for five minutes. Perform the open-loop technique clockwise on both sides of the groin for one minute. In case of varicose veins, use this method and apply the open-loop technique counterclockwise on the bend of the foot as well.

Itching

When people itch all over, the following magnetic treatment is of great value. Brush the body from head to toe with your hands spread out and your thumbs touching each other.

- Front: seven times
- Right arm: seven times
- Back: seven times
- Left arm: seven times

Bringing the Body into Balance

From the back, lightly stroke the head and spine in small, downward semicircles, beginning with the lower back and ending at the head.

Kidneys

The right kidney is positive magnetic in nature. Therefore, you have to place your left hand over the right kidney. The left kidney has a negative charge, so your right hand has to be placed on the left kidney.

Have your friend lie on his stomach. Stand to the side of his head, and let your hands rest on his kidneys. Let the hands rest for two to three minutes, then slowly rotate your hands in the open-loop manner toward the spine. The touch must be very light and do it only for one minute.

Finally, give the nerves on the spine a little twisting motion. For this your touch is a little firmer and moves in a round, circular motion. Let the nerves know that they have to start working again. After repairing wiring in your house, you turn on the switch. It is the same thing here.

This method is used for older folks when they start to bend forward. In fact, it can be used for anyone with poor posture. It is as if something is pulling them forward from inside. Electrically speaking, the wires are mixed up, and the constant shortcut of electricity makes them pull their bodies forward. Try it and you will be happily surprised.

Stomach

Try this method to help the stomach: The middle finger of your left hand rests on the "cup"—the bones in front of the throat. Place the right hand over the stomach. Do not place it flat, but form a cup with your hand. Keep this hollow hand there for 60 seconds, then make small, soft semicircles over the stomach. This is very good for underweight children and adults. Do this once daily for seven days, then two times weekly.

Here is a second method: Have your friend sit on a chair. Stand at his left side. Place your left hand over the stomach so that your fingers touch the gallbladder area. Place your right hand on your friend's back so your hands are opposite each other. That means your right hand is more to his right side rather than to the middle.

Decongest Lungs and Heart

Have your friend lie on his back. You stand at his feet. Softly and slowly stroke both legs from the knees down. Shake your hands to break the magnetic link, then come back in a semicircle to the knees. Do this work for five minutes. Strokes must be featherweight—hardly touching the body—and in a slow, rhythmic motion.

The result in conditions of congested heart and lungs is fabulous.

Sleeplessness

Work in the manner previously described; however, rest over the toes for a second. Then shake your hands and start from the knees down. Do it in slow, rhythmic, soothing strokes.

Nervousness

When your friend is very nervous, do not give foot-compression massage more than once a week. Magneto therapy over the whole body, particularly the soothing spiral, will achieve more satisfying results.

Spleen

The spleen is a very important organ. No wonder God planted it so deeply in our bodies so that nothing can happen to this delicate organ. It is the only organ in the body that has two auras. It is also the only organ to be in complete yin-yang balance.

I have studied every available book on the spleen. A blocked up, congested spleen is a mystery. It is a gland of inner secretion, and once the ducts become congested, we are in severe trouble.

An enlarged spleen (often the result of congestion) is capable of raising the left rib cage visibly. There is very little pain connected with it, but there is fullness and pressure. A sluggish, congested spleen can add to mental instability, depression, and stupor. A congested spleen causes a yellow complexion, and brown discoloration appears over the eyes, cheeks, and around the mouth. It may affect the heartbeat, and often people sigh a lot.

Being afraid of people, cellars, darkness, and closed rooms; or weakness and disorientation can all point to troubles in the spleen. People with spleen trouble seem to be more affected by haunted houses and foreign energy possessions, and many are obsessed or possessed for years until a helping minister or a psychic steps in to release these poor people from their entities.

To open the congested areas of the spleen, stand at the head of your worktable or slightly to the left side of your friend. Place the fingertips of your right hand under the right armpit. Rest your left hand over his/her solar plexus. Hold your hands in this position until you feel heat or throbbing. Your left hand will feel it more distinctly. Watch the color coming into your friend's face. See the lines in the face smoothing out. Watch the dark discoloration go!

Do this work after you have made the parallel and the spiral strokes, and do it seven days in a row. On the second day, the person may expel a sour, putrid stool—black or dark green in color.

Try this simple method on all who are mentally confused, epileptic, or mentally exhausted; and try it on your friends with blood impurities, acne, wrinkles, or discolorations of skin in the face and arms.

The spleen stores the body's electricity. If the spleen is not in order, the brain takes over this job. However, this has a drawback. People become egocentric and accomplish nothing worthwhile.

Lymphatic System

The lymphatic system is greatly helped by Swedish massage. Here is an addition to this work of massage therapy, and you will like it! You do not have to undress your friend. Just loosen his collar.

Sit on the right side of your friend. Place the fingers of your left hand on the cervicals of his neck. The right hand goes under your friend's left armpit.

Now relax and feel. Imagine and direct with your prayers and your mind the proper flow of the lymphatic system. First, the left hand of your friend will become warm. Second, the left foot will be warmer than the right foot. Then the right arm will tingle or become warm. After this, you can interrupt your effort. With strokes, brush down the body—the front for one minute and the back for one minute. This work takes 10 to 15 minutes of your time, but the result is remarkable. Wounds will heal faster. Ulcers on the legs will start to heal. Swollen glands start to disappear as the tissue becomes better nourished and the accumulated waste is better expelled.

The lymphatic fluid is very much under the influence of the magnetic field. Every woman adds three to five pounds of fluid when the moon is full and will lose it one or two days later. Every hyperactive person becomes more hyper when the moon is at its peak. Sleeping pills are used twice as much, and hyperactive children become worse during this time. We just have not paid too much attention to the electromagnetic influence of the environment on our lymphatic fluid. The laying on of hands in the discussed manner will ease many woes in a simple, remarkable way.

Blood

Life is in the blood. The secret power behind the movement of the blood is a great deal of magnetic nature—the movement of each individual blood cell, the disintegration of them, the joining together, the separating, the giving up of energy to each other, the lumping together as in blood clots. Behind all this is electromagnetic power, the secret of the universe, the untapped energies beyond, working in our bloodstream.

The hands directed by the will are the only instruments to direct and correct a faulty magnetic life pattern in the blood. This is the way to influence the faulty electromagnetic pattern when it decides to clot the blood.

Blood Clots

Have your friend lie comfortably on the bed or worktable, with his knees flexed. His hands should be folded as in prayer, but his forefingers should form a pyramid. His thumbs close it. Cover your friend with a light blanket for warmth and comfort. There is nothing like a blanket pulled over you to give you more security. Now sit on your friend's left side. Spread your arms out so the right hand is over his head. The left hand is slipped under the cover. Hold it close to the tailbone. You cuddle your friend visibly and invisibly. Your hands do not touch the body at all but remain one inch away from it.

Now relax and tell your friend to do the same. Concentrate on your work with all your heart. Pray that your energies will be poured into your friend's body. In case someone wants to help you, let him do so by touching your shoulders while standing behind you; in this way, he can also pour energies through you into the patient's body.

Under your hands the miracle takes place. The blood becomes magnetically charged, and the blood clot disintegrates. Visibly, the redness disappears. Also, the breathing becomes easier, and the fever disappears. (The credit for this method goes to Rev. Dr. F. M. Houston.) The following story will illustrate the efficacy of this method.

I was invited to a party. I enjoy parties most when I can sit aside and observe the happiness of others. So I did. A huge man turned to me and out of the blue sky told me that he was a physicist. Then he said, "Please tell me what I can do for myself. I do not feel well."

We sat down, and in a second, the Lord showed me that this man had a blood clot just in front of his heart, ready to loosen any minute. I didn't know what to say or how to say it, but help came when the man said, "I did not want to come to this party, but an inner voice told me to come."

Now I knew that this man was a "sensitive," so I fully told him what the Lord had revealed to me. "I will look for myself," he said. Then he closed his eyes. When he opened them, he stared at me and said, "There is a clot in front of my heart. What can I do?"

Now it was my turn to ask questions, and I found out that this man was America's most outstanding scientist as well as a top psychic researcher. Often he was called to psychic conferences overseas.

We found a quiet room, and I performed the described magnetic healing on him. Wonder of wonders, this beautiful soul could describe every detail that was going on. He said, "The light from the right hand is blue and white. It separates the lumped-together blood cells. Now it comes closer to the problem area. It chisels away at the problem. First the outsides become light. The blood clot starts to disappear. It disappears like a mist when the sun is coming through." In this moment, the scientist took a deep breath—his huge chest expanded, then fell back to normal.

I am the luckiest person on Earth to have had such an opportunity to meet a man who could see—actually see and not guess—what was taking place. Thank God for this.

To Stop Bleeding

To stop bleeding, you sit at the right side of your patient. Cradle him by holding your left hand over the head, and the right hand under the tailbone.

A young physician was drafted during the Vietnam War. When he said goodbye, I had an intuition to tell him how to stop bleeding electromagnetically. Two years passed before he returned, a quiet, serene, changed person. "Your advice on how to stop bleeding has saved many soldiers," he stated. "We hardly lost anyone, even in severe injuries and severed arms and legs. It helped." Without great danger and losses, the soldiers could be sent back to hospitals in excellent shape.

Infection

Use these methods to stop infections:

- Break the impact of viral infections by using deep and steady pressure with hands over the bottom of the right rib cage and over both sides of the chest.
- Break polio infection next to the shoulder blades. I often use a light karate stroke on congestions near the shoulder blades.
- Use Dr. Houston's method for strep infections described in his helpful book, *The Healing Benefits of Acupressure.*

The Common Cold

The common cold responds favorably to magneto therapy. Have your friend stand or sit. Your right hand lightly touches the spot between his shoulder blades. After 60 seconds, rub his back with the spiral movement previously described. The spirals must be large and cover the width of his back. Do it with your right hand. Have the left hand resting on the throat or forehead.

Pneumonia

When the cold has already settled in the lungs and pneumonia is imminent or already there, the following method of laying on hands has saved many, many people.

Place your cupped right hand on the forehead so that the little finger still touches the bridge of the nose. Your left hand cradles the back of the head. Sit comfortably because this will take 10 to 15 minutes. You will hear the congestion break up in the lungs. After that, place your right hand on your friend's chest, the left hand on his back, and finish this work with another five minutes of your hands.

For all head congestions, headaches, and nervous disorders, you place the opposite hand (left) on the forehead and the right hand on the back of the head and rest it there another three minutes.

Sunburn and Other Burns

For several minutes, perform light parallel strokes, but do not touch the skin. Also, when the skin is subject to cold and partially frozen, this procedure brings life back into it.

Bruises and Other Injuries

Sometimes after someone has broken his leg or arm, has been bandaged and has had the bandage removed, the pain still exists. There are two methods to help. The first method is to use lengthwise strokes over the injured area but not touching anything. The second method (American Indian) is to place the middle finger of your right hand beneath the skull of your friend. With the left hand, lightly touch the injured limb or other injured part.

All bruises and other injuries respond most favorably to both methods.

Exhaustion

Place a piece of cotton cloth or handkerchief over the person (who is fully clothed). Bring your lips close and firmly right under the heart (tip of heart) and bring "life-breath" into the exhausted person for over one minute. Life-breath is performed by taking a deep breath and, with the mouth shaped in an "o," quickly expel the breath in a puff directed at the desired location. Eighteen breaths are needed. The entire blood will be magnetized with life-breath.

Give an overly excited person life-breath over the stomach where the sternum ends. Soon the excitement will be gone.

The life-breath method is also indicated for fainting spells, convulsions, and electroshock therapies. Give aid by lowering the patient's head when pale, or lifting the head when red. Then make 20 quick, lengthwise strokes. After that, give life-breath to both heart and stomach.

Inability to Concentrate and Emotional Instability

Remember that the lack of concentration in children can be caused by neglecting to cut their fingernails. Fingernails that are too long have a tendency to hinder the electromagnetic forces. These forces easily back up and become destructive to the concentration and the development of the inner being of the child.

Women with overly long fingernails have trouble keeping calm and being steady in mood and balance, and they are easily upset and lacking in electromagnetic energy in general.

❧ CHAPTER NINE ❧

Collection of Knowledge

This chapter contains an odd collection of knowledge gathered over the years. I hope that you enjoy reading it as much as I enjoyed compiling it.

Solomon's Song (Solomon 4:14)

Use the following procedure every month to cleanse and take impurities out of the body.

1 tsp. spikenard
2 pinches saffron
$1/4$ tsp. calamus
2 sticks cinnamon
$1/4$ tsp. frankincense
$1/4$ tsp. myrrh
$1/4$ tsp. aloes

In approximately seven cups purified water, add herbs and boil 15 minutes, simmer, put in a glass jar, and refrigerate. Drink two cups daily for three days. Do this once a month to cleanse and remove impurities from the body.

Reading Body Signals

Left ankle swelling: Heart problem
Right ankle swelling: Kidney problem

Sprained ankle:	Emotionally ungrounded
Large hips:	Pituitary gland
Overmuscular legs:	Rigid personality; will not change easily; firm in beliefs
Undermuscular legs:	Depends on others for support
Right shoulder pain:	First heart chamber trouble
Left shoulder pain:	Entire heart is in trouble
Throat problems:	Liver problems
Continued sore throat:	Restrained anger
Stiff neck:	Prolonged tension
Hemorrhoids:	Liver problem; holding on to all feelings too long and too tight—let go

Taste or Appetite Changes As Warning Signals

If you notice an unusual, persistent change in your taste or appetite, it may be nature's way of warning you that something is wrong with your body. Here are descriptions of the more common changes in taste and appetite and of the problems that may underlie them.

- Sour taste, or a persistent craving for tart fruits, may indicate difficulties with the gallbladder or liver.

- Bitter taste may suggest vitamin and mineral deficiencies, or colitis.

- Craving for sweets may signal the development of hypoglycemia or diabetes, not enough protein, or Candida albicans infection.

- Craving for spicy foods may indicate difficulties in the lungs or sinuses.

- Dislike for meat or taste loss may indicate cellular distress and possibly cancer. Many stomach cancers are associated with the symptoms of unpleasant taste and a dislike for meat. This may also be caused by a lack of hydrochloric acid. Taste loss may indicate a zinc deficiency.

An occasional craving or unusual taste is no cause for alarm. However, if the change is persistent, bring it to the attention of your physician.

Eyes

Your amazing eyes do more than just see. They can reveal important things about your health, experts say.

- If one pupil is larger than the other, it can indicate that a tumor is hidden somewhere in the body.
- Red eyes can signal an infection in the eyes that is usually caused by a virus or bacteria. Red eyes can also be caused by allergies or air pollution.
- Changes in vision, such as being able to see better on one day than another or seeing double, are warning signs of diabetes. If you already know you're a diabetic and experience these symptoms, it may mean the disease has not been properly controlled.
- If the whites of the eyes turn yellow, it can be a sign of hepatitis, a blockage of the gallbladder duct, or the presence of a tumor in the pancreas.
- Difficulty reading, even while wearing the correct glasses, may point to thyroid trouble.
- Being able to see better on cloudy days or in the evenings than on bright, sunny days—or seeing a rainbow or halo around glowing streetlights—are possible signs of glaucoma.
- Vision that wavers between clear and blurry can be an indication of high blood pressure.

Don't treat yourself. Let a competent medical authority confirm the problem.

Seven Pulses for the Westerner

1. Lazy—weak or dropped kidney
2. Pounding—artery hepatic
3. Wiry—inflammation
4. Fast—coxalgia plexus
5. Intermittent—phrenic nerve
6. Pounding with expansion—abdominal aorta
7. Jumping—pancreas and liver

Legs

If the left leg is short, take a cloth drenched with vinegar. Place it over your forehead, and the leg straightens out at once. If the right leg is short, place soda on the forehead. Reason: The sympathetic nervous system is supposed to be alkaline, and the parasympathetic nervous system should be acid. If this is not in order, the length of the legs will change.

To recognize an acid condition: Look for dehydration, a lump in the throat, and dry skin.

To recognize an alkaline condition: Look for itching, stiffness, night cough, night cramps, sensitivity, and overweight below the waist.

Scientific Breathing: A Time-Saver

To strengthen breathing, try the following methods.

Lower abdominal breathing:
Make circles of the index fingers and thumbs and extend other fingers straight out and close together. Place hands palms down on groin. Elbows should be at right angles to your body. Breathe deeply. The breath will be confined to the area below the navel.

Intercostal breathing:
Make circles of index fingers and thumbs and fold remaining fingers into the palm. Place hands palms down on groin. Elbows should be at right angles to your body. Breathe deeply. This breath will be felt in the lower abdomen and up to the area under the ribs.

Utilizing upper clavicular area of lungs:
Make baby's fists by folding four fingers on each hand over thumbs. Place fists on groin and breathe deeply and slowly. This breath will fill your entire lungs.

What Amino Acids Do

Histidine:
Pineal—right and left side
Pancreas—right and left side

Aspartic acid:
Pineal—right and left side

Asparagine:
Pancreas—right and left side

Tyrosine:
Lower jawbone

Isoleucine:
Heart
Left side

Serine:
Lung—right side

Proline:
Liver—left side

Methionine:
Liver—right side

Glycine:
Kidney—right and left side

Lysine:
Spleen

Homocystine:
Pineal—right and left side

Leucine:
Pancreas—right and left side
Elbows

Tryptophan + Carnosine:
Pancreas—right and left side

Phenylalanine:
Liver
Jawbone—left side
Vagina—right and left side

Glutamic acid:
Lung—left side
Brain—right side

Cystine:
Liver—left side

Alanine:
Liver—left side

Gamma-aminobutyric acid:
Kidney—right and left side

Hydroxylysine + Norvaline:
Spleen—right and left side

Coffee

Personally, I am not in favor of coffee. However, I am asked over and over what coffee does. Like every plant, it does something to the system. What follows is a list you might enjoy reading. Do not use milk in coffee because it crystallizes, causing gallstones, kidney stones, and hardening of the arteries.

Sugar in coffee is also a no-no. But a little bit of honey in coffee makes the difference. When I need an extra lift after ten hours of work and I have to be alert for another four hours, I take half a cup of coffee with a little honey in it, and zoom, I can go!

It is also important to know, when taking coffee enemas, what kind of coffee will do what. All coffee beans stimulate the pineal and pituitary, and they are extra good in enemas when cancer is present. Some coffee beans stimulate the spleen, and some stimulate the pancreas.

Always remember, a little coffee goes a long way. It can be a strong remedy if chosen properly.

Coffee Beans	Affected Area
Colombian:	To rectum—up to stomach gland—to heart (extra good)
Guatemalan:	To rectum—to pineal—to coccyx—vitamin B_6
Mexican maragogipe:	To duodenum—pepsin—pineal
Kenyan:	Pancreas—grape sugar
Hawaiian Kona:	Kidney-beryllium
New Guinean:	Spleen—sex (male/female)—folic acid
Mexican:	Pineal—cortisone to heart—cystine—iron
Peruvian:	Larynx
Salvadoran:	Tongue—borax soda—quartz crystal
Continental roast:	Appendix—gypsum—calcium
Viennese roast:	Pituitary—cobalt—quartz—salt
Colombian supreme:	Pineal—gray lime—insulin
Jamaican:	Pineal—liver—heart—element B_2
Costa Rican:	Liver—manganese—B_{12}
Nicaraguan:	Pineal—magnesium—citric acid—vitamin E
Mocha:	Pineal—bone ash—iron—cobalt

Java:	Colon and rectum—vitamin C—digitalis—lime phosphate
Ethiopian:	Liver—radiation mineral
	Liver—electrical magnetic
Indian:	Spleen

SPECIFIC HEALING PROPERTIES IN FOODS

Anise:	For flatulent conditions.
Apples:	Whatever ails you: gallbladder trouble, liver trouble, diarrhea, tooth decay, constipation, loss of appetite; good as poultices, too. When someone is very ill, take an apple and scrape the meat with a silver spoon. You will see them get better.
Apricots:	To detoxify the liver and pancreas.
Asparagus:	For fatty tumors and the like. Helpful in urinary secretions.
Avocado:	A fat and protein supplier. Good for the diabetic.
Barley:	A calcium supplier, colon aid, and lymph cleanser.
Beans (adzuki):	For kidney trouble and swollen ankles.
Beans (green):	Remove metallic poison. Good for the malfunctions of the pancreas.
Beans (lima):	Make a dish with lima beans, bell peppers, and sweet potato to combat drug residue.
Beans (red):	Build muscles. Served with corn, a complete protein.
Beans (white):	For the eyes and for liver trouble.
Beans and corn:	Muscle builders (especially red beans).
Beef:	Muscle food.
Beets:	Spleen food.
Bell pepper:	Eyes and digestion (increases pepsin).
Black bean juice:	For hoarseness and laryngitis.
Blackberries:	Colon food. For diarrhea.
Blackstrap molasses:	A mineral and iron supplier.
Blueberries:	Pancreas food. For sugar problems.
Blueberry and banana:	Pancreatitis.
Buckwheat:	For energy and warmth. For strong muscles.

Butternut:	Liver food.
Cabbage:	For vitamin U, the tissue builder.
Carrots:	Eyes, Blood, and lymph.
Celery:	A low-calorie reducing aid.
Celery seed:	Drink the tea for obesity.
Cherries:	For gout.
Cherries (sour):	For gout and as a blood cleanser.
Chicken:	A gland food.
Chickpeas:	A gland food. Good protein. An antiviral, particularly antipolio virus.
Crab apple:	For vertigo.
Cranberry:	A kidney food. Releases sudden cramps, as in asthma and the like.
Cucumber:	A skin remedy, kidney cleanser, and infection cleanser.
Currants:	Build resistance to colds. For anemia.
Eggplant:	Give the peelings and dulse to the afflicted tumor.
Figs:	A dewormer.
Fish:	Good protein and iodine supplier.
Garlic:	Carbohydrate residue in tissue and glands.
Grapefruit:	A lime supplier. A flu destroyer.
Grapes:	Antitumor; good for anemia; an aura builder.
Indian corn:	Perfect food for humans—has all the energies, amino acids, and hormones the body needs.
Kale:	For resistance to colds.
Leek:	For reducing; a pancreas food, tissue builder, and brain food.
Lemon:	Vitamin C.
Lemon (white of rind):	Bioflavonoid. Strengthens tissue.
Lentils:	Iron. Contains protein supplies of the best quality.
Lime:	For yellow jaundice.
Meat:	Lots of calories. Protein that gives an explosive energy. Appetite satisfying.
Millet:	Meat of the vegetarian. Fifteen percent protein.
Oats:	Brain food.
Oils, cold-pressed:	Needed to assimilate the proteins from vegetables. Also a kidney food.

Okra:	Regulates female bleeding. Gives strength to leukemia patients.
Okra and apples:	For ulceration of the stomach.
Onion:	Make a soup of fresh red and white onions and collards for the flu.
Oranges:	Vitamin C for flu prevention.
Papaya:	For protein digestion.
Parsley:	For piles.
Parsley root:	For kidneys. When boiled in white wine, it is for the heart.
Parsnip:	For intolerance to milk.
Peaches:	Good during pregnancy.
Pears:	Kidney and colon.
Peas:	Green and dried peas are good sources of protein and good for weak stomachs.
Pineapple:	Enzyme supplier.
Pomegranate:	A dewormer.
Potatoes (red):	For stomach and duodenal ulcer.
Potato peelings:	For kidney ailments.
Prunes:	Iron, constipation.
Pumpkin:	Spleen and pancreas food.
Pumpkin seeds:	Dewormer, parasites.
Radishes:	In small amounts, promote bile flow.
Raisin:	Anemia; blood builder.
Rhubarb:	Colon cleanser.
Rice:	Universal acceptance by all tissues (overrated at the present time).
Rice gruel:	Diarrhea.
Romaine lettuce:	Viral infection.
Rutabaga:	Food for prayer. Feeds friendly bacteria in colon. Once a week it would be good.
Rye:	Muscle builder.
Sauerkraut:	Keeps old folks' ailments away.
Sesame seeds:	Complete amino acid supplier. Make strong-willed people. Supplies osmium, a trace mineral.
Spinach:	Good for you if you have anemia.
Strawberries:	A skin berry.

Strawberries *and squash:*	Remove metallic poisons, especially arsenic.
Sunflower seeds:	Feeds eyes, sinuses, and glands.
Sweet potato:	Gland food.
Swiss chard:	Arthritis (contains Wulzen factor).
Tomato:	As poultices in deep-rooted afflictions. When stewed, good for liver. Fresh tomatoes are a vitamin C supplier. Green tomatoes in very small quantities are a gland stimulant. Always remove the core of the stem. Make a deep insertion. This stem part is poisonous.
Turnips:	For deep-rooted tumors. For deep-rooted resentments.
Watercress:	Supplier of vitamins C and E.
Watermelon:	For sluggish kidney; a kidney cleanser.
Wheat:	Starch and calorie supplier.
Yams:	Hormone food.
Yogurt:	Intestinal health.

⟆ Recommended Reading ⟅

The following books are available at Hanna's Herb Shop:
5684 Valmont Rd., Boulder, CO 80301 • (800) 206-6722

The Healing Benefits of Acupressure,
by Rev. Dr. Fred M. Houston, D.C.

Fluoride: The Aging Factor,
by John Yiamouyiannis

The Yeast Connection,
by Dr. W. Crook

Fight Back Against Arthritis,
by Dr. Robert Bingham

About the Author

Hanna Kroeger was born of German Christian missionaries. She studied nursing at the University of Freiburg, Germany, and worked in a hospital for natural healing under Professor Brauchle. In 1953, she and her family came to America.

After coming to the United States, Hanna took advantage of the education offered in this country, ranging from Amerindian herbology to massage. She obtained a doctorate of metaphysics (MsD), and became an ordained minister in the Universal Church of the Masters, a church well known for its work in contact and spiritual healing. Besides writing, teaching, and lecturing, she established a health food store in Boulder, Colorado; as well as a health resort, the Peaceful Meadow Retreat, where her knowledge of nutrition is used with exciting results.

Other Hay House Titles of Related Interest

Aromatherapy A–Z,
by Connie and Alan Higley, and Pat Leatham

Aura Soma—Healing Through Color, Plant, and Crystal Energy,
by Irene Dalichow and Mike Booth

Deep Healing—The Essence of Mind/Body Medicine,
by Emmett Miller, M.D.

The Essential Flower Essence Handbook, by Lila Devi

Heal Your Body, by Louise L. Hay

Heal Your Life with Home Remedies and Herbs, by Hanna Kroeger

Healing with Herbs and Home Remedies A–Z, by Hanna Kroeger

Prostate Health in 90 Days, by Larry Clapp, Ph.D., J.D.

The Roots of Healing, by Andrew Weil, M.D.,
and Others, with Michael Toms

(All of the above are available at your local bookstore,
or may be ordered by calling Hay House at 800-654-5126.)

We hope you enjoyed this Hay House book. If you would like to receive a free catalog featuring additional Hay House books and products, or if you would like information about the Hay Foundation, please contact:

Hay House, Inc.
P.O. Box 5100
Carlsbad, CA 92018-5100

(760) 431-7695 or **(800) 654-5126**
(760) 431-6948 (fax) or **(800) 650-5115 (fax)**

Please visit the Hay House Website at: **www.hayhouse.com**